Biochemical and Biological Studies on Oleuropein and Its Hypoglycemic Effect

I0503540

A Thesis Submitted to the Department of Chemistry College
of Science of Baghdad University as Partial Fulfillment of
Requirements for the Degree of Doctor of
Philosophy in Clinical Biochemistry

By

Hasan Fayadh Samir Al-Azzawi

B.Sc. Chemistry 1981
M.Sc. Clinical Chemistry 1986

SUPERVISED BY

PROF. DR. SAMI AL-MUDHAFFAR

Ph.D.Biochemistry

1425 A.H   2004 A.D

Supervisor Certification

I certify that this thesis was prepared under my supervision at the University of Baghdad as a partial requirement for the Degree of Doctor of Philosophy in clinical Biochemistry.

Signature:

Supervisor: Professor Dr. Sami Al-Mudhaffar

Date:

Chairman of the postgraduate studies Recommendation:

In view of the available certifications, I forward this thesis for debate by the examining.

Signature:

Name: **Prof. Suad.Al-Araji**

Chairman of the postgraduate studies/College of Science, Chemistry Department

Date:

Committee Certification

We certify that we read this thesis and as examining committee examined the student in its content, and that in our opinion it is adequate with () standing as a thesis for the Degree of Doctor of Philosophy in clinical Biochemistry.

Signature:

Name: **Prof. Yousif Ali Al-Fattahie**

Date:

(Chairman)

Signature:

Name: Prof.Ali M. Hasan

Date:

(Member)

Signature:

Name Prof.: Hathama R.Hasan

Date:

(Member)

Signature:

Name: **Prof. Ferah.G.Al-Salihi**

Date:

(Member)

Signature:

Name: Prof. Khalid. S. Al-Delymie

Date:

(Member)

Signature:

Name: Prof. Sami Al-Mudhaffar

Date:

(Supervisor)

Approved for the Council of the College of Science

Signature:

Name*:* Prof. A. M. Taleb

(Dean of the College of Science)

Date:

Acknowledgments

I wish to express my deepest gratitude to my supervisor ***Dr.Sami Al-Mudhaffar*** for his encouragement to start this work and for the opportunity to be a member of the inspiring research group. His endless support and constructive criticism has been precious during these years.

I owe my thanks to Assistant Professor ***Dr.Gabbar Al-Hadithai,*** Head of the Department of basic science, college of agriculture university of Baghdad, for providing the facilities for my work in his department and for his support.

My thanks go to ***Dr. Hazim Al-Salhi***, Head of the Department of clinical Chemistry at Military Rashid hospital for providing the facilities for technical assistance in carrying out a part of this study.

I am grateful to workers in Central medical laboratory, Biological control center and College of medicine at Nahrain University for technical help in carrying out a part of this study.

My friends in the Departments of Physiology and Clinical Nutrition in College of Veterinary medicine deserve warm thanks, for making my work easier during these years, for giving hand in solving problems, and for providing a pleasant working atmosphere.

My special thanks go to my brother ***Mohamed Saiel Alhamdani*** from the College of Pharmacy, Department of Clinical Biochemistry for his technical assistance in preparing the manuscript of this work.

I am deeply indebted to **Prof. Visioli** at University of Milan (Italy) for the valuable discussion and helpful comments and to my friend Aimer H.Alyuass,Adanan M. for NMR measurements and to My brother Dr.Sami . F. at Garish University (Jordan) for his assistance in literature review.

My warmest thanks belong to my parents for their confidence in me and for being always so supportive and interested in my work and well-being. I would like to thank them. Finally, my dearest thanks are addressed to my family, my wife for her love and tireless support, and our wonderful and active sons *Noor*, *Sanna* and *Aula* for being the sunshine of my life

Hassan. Al-Azzawi
September 2004

Name of student: Assistant Prof. Hasan Fayadh Samir Al-Azzawie.

Name of Supervisor: Prof. Sami Al-Mudhaffar.

Thesis Title: Biochemical and biological studies on Oleuropein and its hypoglycemic effect.

Abstract

The phenolic compounds of three common *olea europeae* variety leaves, grown in different areas of Iraq (Labeeb, Al-Asharsy and Manzanillo) were studied using different methods of extraction, isolation and purification by thin layer chromatography (TLC) and high pressure liquid chromatography (HPLC). The dried olive leaves were extracted with methanol: water (1:1 v/v) or ethanol: water (3:1 v/v) until complete extraction of phenolic compounds had been achieved. The methanolic extract was then conducted to dryness, re-dissolved in methanol and analyzed by TLC and RP-HPLC. There was no difference in qualitative phenolic profiles but, different levels of oleuropein were observed in these different varieties. The polyphenols that detected in olive leaf extract were: hydroxytyrosol, tyrosol, hydroxytyrosol glucoside, caffeic acid, elenolic acid derivatives, verbascoside, rutin, luteolin 7-O glucoside, and apigenin 7-O glucoside.

The recovery of oleuropein was compared between acid and base extraction. Quantitative data of the levels of phenolic compounds were obtained by the different procedures. The oleuropein was significantly affected by both acid and base treatment, resulted in the liberation of hydroxytyrosol. The levels of hydroxytyrosol produced after 24 hour of acid treatment were 50 times than produced by base treatment.

The major phenolic compounds of olive leaves extract were examined and found to be capable of inhibition of low density lipoprotein peroxidation at optimal doses to have remarkable biological activity contributing to that previously reported for the major phenolic compounds. Oleuropein activity was 49% of mean protection.

Oleuropein and its metabolites, oleuropein aglycone, hydroxytyrosol were compared with vitamin E regard to their antioxidant activity by kinetic studies in a model system. Oleuropein and hydroxytyrosol were much more efficient than vitamin E as antioxidant. The methanolic extract of olive leaves was shown to have inhibitory effects on the hemolysis of rabbit erythrocytes induced by 2, 2-azo-bis-2-amidinopropane (APPH). Oleuropein exhibited strong antioxidant efficiency against hemolysis of erythrocytes induced by free radicals.

Oleuropein and its metabolites isolated from olive leaves extract were examined *in vitro* for their antimicrobial activity against five different species of pathogenic bacteria isolated from human patients (*E.coli; H.influenza; salmonella typhi; staph. aureus* and *K.pneumonia*. The results obtained indicated that all of the phenolic compounds except oleuropein glucoside had antimicrobial activity against all bacterial strains.

Oleuropein was tested for its blood glucose lowering activity in rabbits and showed a dose dependent prophylactic effect against the rise of blood glucose induced by alloxan. Best results were obtained at a dose of 100 mg/kg of the oleuropein. In the rabbits that rendered hyperglycemia by alloxan for 16 weeks, and then treated with a dose of 20 mg pure oleuropein daily for further 16 weeks, normalization of the blood glucose was observed.

The effect of the daily intake of 20 mg pure oleuropein in alloxan induced diabetic rabbits on lipid profile, uric acid, glycated hemoglobin, erythrocyte enzymatic antioxidant activity Superoxide dismutase (SOD), Glutathione reductase (GRx), Glutathione peroxidase (GPx), Glucose-6-phosphodehydrogenase (G-6PD), and glutathione (GSH) content, as well as non enzymatic antioxidant levels (vitamin C, vitamin E and β-carotene) in addition to parameters of oxidative stress, thiobarbituric acid reactant substances, and total antioxidant capacity were carried out in two parallel routes: alloxan induced diabetic rabbits administrated 20 mg of oleuropein daily for 16 weeks period and NIDDM patients administrated 1.0 gm of oleuropein daily for 6 months period. Significant changes in all parameters were observed.

Binding of I-^{125} insulin to intact human lymphocytes isolated from non insulin dependent diabetes mellitus patients was studied. The binding characteristics were studied and analyzed by scatchard plot. There was a high order low capacity binding sites with an affinity constant of 2×10^{9} M^{-1} and a low order, high capacity binding sties with an affinity constant of 1.4×10^{9} M^{-1}. The number of binding sites was significantly reduced in non-insulin dependent diabetes mellitus patients against healthy subjects. Long term administration of 1.0 gm of pure oleuropein daily for 6 months was associated with improvement in binding percent, protected the insulin receptors from oxidative damage, maintaining its functional integrity, and increase in both order of binding sites although no significant change in affinity constant was observed.

Finally the present study investigated for the first time the effect of oleuropein on histological changes possibly occurring in islets of Langerhans in pancreatic alloxan induced diabetic mice. Islets of Langerhans showed continuous hypertrophy with hyperplasia, lymphocyte infiltration and a significant increase in the average of islets diameter, while treatment with pure oleuropein showed a decrease average islet diameter with few small islets were atrophoid as a result of oleuropein intake, all of islets appeared normal as of the control animals.

List of Contents

Content	Pages
List of contents	I
List of Figures	VI
List of Tables	VIII
List of Abbreviation	XII
Summary	XV

Chapter One: Introduction and Literature Review

Chapter Three: Results and Dissuasion

List of Figures

3-19	Levels of high density lipoprotein (Mean ± SD) in healthy and alloxan induced diabetic rabbits after long term administration of 20 mg oleuropein daily for l6 weeks.	132
3-20	Levels of high density lipoprotein (Mean ± SD) in healthy subjects and non insulin dependent diabetic mellitus patients after long term administration of 1.0 gm oleuropein daily for 6 months	133
3-21	Levels of low density lipoprotein (Mean ± SD) in healthy and alloxan diabetic rabbits after long administration of 20 mg oleuropein daily for 16 weeks.	135
3-22	Levels of low density lipoprotein (Mean ± SD) in healthy subjects and non insulin dependent diabetic mellitus patients after long administration of 1.0 gm oleuropein daily for 6 months.	135
3-23	Levels of very low density lipoprotein (Mean ± SD) in healthy and alloxan diabetic rabbits after long term administration of 20 mg oleuropein daily for l6 weeks.	136
3-24	Levels of very low density lipoprotein (Mean ± SD) in healthy subjects and non insulin dependent diabetic mellitus patients after long term administration of 1.0 gm oleuropein daily for 6 months.	136
3-25	Levels of serum triglycerides (Mean ± SD) in healthy and alloxan diabetic rabbits after long administration of 20 mg oleuropein daily for l6 weeks	137
3-26	Levels of serum triglycerides (Mean ±SD) in healthy subjects and non insulin dependent diabetic mellitus patients after long administration of 1.0 gm oleuropein daily for 6 months.	137
3-27	Levels of serum uric acid (Mean ± SD) in healthy and alloxan diabetic rabbits after long administration of 20 mg oleuropein daily for 16 weeks.	141
3-28	Levels of serum uric acid (Mean ± SD) in healthy subjects and non insulin dependent diabetic mellitus patients after long administration of 1.0 gm oleuropein daily for 6 months.	141
3-29	Levels of glycated hemoglobin (Mean ± SD) in healthy and alloxan diabetic rabbits after long term administration of 20 mg oleuropein daily for l6 weeks.	142
3-30	Levels of glycated hemoglobin (Mean ± SD) in healthy subjects and non insulin dependent diabetic mellitus patients after long term administration of 1.0 gm oleuropein daily for 6 months.	142
3-31	Levels of malondialdehyde (Mean ± SD) in erythrocytes of healthy and alloxan diabetic rabbits patients after long term administration of 20 mg oleuropein daily for l6 weeks.	145
3-32	Levels of malondialdehyde (Mean ±SD) in erythrocytes of healthy subjects and non insulin dependent diabetic mellitus patients after long term administration of 1.0 gm oleuropein daily for 6 months	145
3-33	Levels of plasma malondialdehyde (Mean ± SD) in healthy and alloxan diabetic rabbits after long term administration of 20 mg oleuropein daily for l6 weeks.	145
3-34	Levels of plasma malondialdehyde (Mean ± SD) in healthy subjects and non insulin dependent diabetic mellitus patients after long term administration of 1.0 gm oleuropein daily for 6 months	145

X

List of Abbreviations

ABTS	2,2-azo-bis(3-ethylbenzothiazoline-6-sulphonate)
4CL	4-coumarate: coenzyme A ligase
AAPH	2,2-azo-bis-(2-amidinopropane)
AGE_S	Advance glycosylation end products
APCI	Atmospheric pressure chemical ionisation
API	Atmospheric pressure ionization
API-MS	Atmospheric pressure ionization – mass spectrometry
APPI	Atmospheric pressure photoionization
B	Bound
CA4H	Cinnamic acid 4-hydroxylase
CAT	Catalase
CBG	Cytosolic β -glucosidase
CDNB	Chloro-dinitrobenzene
CE	High performance capillary electrophoresis
CETP	Cholesterol ester transfer protein
CHD	Coronary heart disease
CID	Collision-induced dissociation
COMT	Catechol-O-methyltransferase
CPM	Count per minute
D.W	Distilled water
DAD	Diode array detection
DTNB	Dithiobisnitrobenzoic acid
DPPH	2,2-diphenyl-1-picrylhydrazyl
EA	Elenolic acid
EC	Electrochemical
ESI	Electrospray ionization
ESI-MS	Electrospray ionisation – mass spectrometry
EtOH	Ethanol
ETP	Ester transfer protein
F	Free
G-6-PD	Glucose-6-phosphoatedehydrogenase
GAE	Gallic acid equivalent
GC-MS	Gas chromatography – mass spectrometry
GH4C1 cells	Cultivated cells from rat pituitary gland, clone 1
GLUT4	Glucose transporter
GPx	Glutathione peroxidase
GRx	Glutathione reductase
GSH	Glutathione reduced
GSSG	Glutathione oxidized
HbA_{1c}	Glycated hemoglobin
HDL-c	High density lipoprotein cholesterol
HHDP	Hexahydroxydiphenoyl
HPLC	high-performance liquid chromatography
HT	Hydroxytyrosol
IC	Inhibition concentration
IDDM	Insulin dependent diabetes mellitus
IE	Ionisation energy

iNOS	Induced nitric oxide synthase
I_0	Intensity of incident light
IR	Infra red
ISI	Ion spray ionization
KRB	Krebs-Ringer bicarbonate
LACT	Lecithin cholesterol acyl transferase
LC	Liquid chromatography
LC-MS	Liquid chromatography – mass spectrometry
LDL-c	Low density lipoprotein cholesterol
LPH	Lactose phlorizine hydrolase
LPL	Lipoprotein lipase
LPS	Lipopolysassharides
m/z	Mass/charge ratio
MBC	Minimum bactericidal concentration
MDA	Malondialdehyde
MeOH	Methanol
MIC	Minimum inhibitory concentration
MP	Mean protection
MPA	Meta-Phosphoric acid
MPLC	Medium pressure liquid chromatography
MS	Mass spectrometry
NADPH	Nicotinamide adenine dinucleotide phosphate (reduced form)
NBT	Nitro blue tetrazolium salt
NIDDM	Non insulin dependent diabetes mellitus
NMR	Nuclear magnetic resonance spectroscopy
NSB	Non specific binding
OD	Optical density
ODS	Octadecylsilane
OFG	Orange Fuchsin Green
OLE	Oleuropein
OLEa	Oleuropein aglycone
Ox-LDL	Oxidized low density lipoprotein
PA	Proton affinity
PAL	Phenylalanine ammonialyase
PBS	Phosphate buffer saline
PCA	Principal component analysis
PDA	Photo-diode array detection
RBC	Red blood cells
RP-HPLC	Reversed phase HPLC
S/N	Signal to noise
SD	Standard deviation
SID	Source-induced dissociation
SOD	Superoxide dismutase
SPE	Solid phase extraction
TBARS	Thiobarbituric acid reactive species
TBA	Thiobarbituric acid
TBHQ	Tert-butylhydroquinone
TEAC	Total equivalent antioxidant capacity

THF	Tetrahydrofuran
TIC	Total ion chromatogram
TLC	Thin layer chromatography
UDPGT	UDP glucuronide transferase
UV/VIS	Ultraviolet / visible
VLDL	Very low density lipoprotein cholesterol
μ	Micron

Summary

The phenolic compounds of three common *olea europeae* variety leaves, grown in different areas of Iraq (Labeeb, Al-Asharsy and Manzanillo) were studied using different methods of extraction, isolation and purification by thin layer chromatography (TLC) and high pressure liquid chromatography (HPLC). The dried olive leaves were extracted with methanol: water (1:1 v/v) or ethanol: water (3:1 v/v) until complete extraction of phenolic compounds had been achieved. The methanolic extract was then conducted to dryness, re-dissolved in methanol and analyzed by TLC and RP-HPLC. There was no difference in qualitative phenolic profiles but, different levels of oleuropein were observed in these different varieties. The polyphenols that detected in olive leaf extract were: hydroxytyrosol, tyrosol, hydroxytyrosol glucoside, caffeic acid, elenolic acid derivatives, verbascoside, rutin, luteolin 7-O glucoside, and apigenin 7-O glucoside.

The recovery of oleuropein was compared between acid and base extraction. Quantitative data of the levels of phenolic compounds were obtained by the different procedures. The oleuropein was significantly affected by both acid and base treatment, resulted in the liberation of hydroxytyrosol. The levels of hydroxytyrosol produced after 24 hour of acid treatment were 50 times than produced by base treatment.

The major phenolic compounds of olive leaves extract were examined and found to be capable of inhibition of low density lipoprotein peroxidation at optimal doses to have remarkable biological activity contributing to that previously reported for the major phenolic compounds. Oleuropein activity was 49% of mean protection.

Oleuropein and its metabolites, oleuropein aglycone, hydroxytyrosol were compared with vitamin E regard to their antioxidant activity by kinetic studies in a model system. Oleuropein and hydroxytyrosol were much more efficient than vitamin E as antioxidant.

The methanolic extract of olive leaves was shown to have inhibitory effects on the hemolysis of rabbit erythrocytes induced by 2, 2-azo-bis-2-amidinopropane (APPH). Oleuropein exhibited strong antioxidant efficiency against hemolysis of erythrocytes induced by free radicals.

Oleuropein and its metabolites isolated from olive leaves extract were examined *in vitro* for their antimicrobial activity against five different species of pathogenic bacteria isolated from human patients (*E.coli; H.influenza; salmonella typhi; staph. aureus* and *K.pneumonia*. The results obtained indicated that all of the phenolic compounds except oleuropein glucoside had antimicrobial activity against all bacterial strains.

Oleuropein was tested for its blood glucose lowering activity in rabbits and showed a dose dependent prophylactic effect against the rise of blood glucose induced by alloxan. Best results were obtained at a dose of 100 mg/kg of the oleuropein. In the rabbits that rendered hyperglycemia by alloxan for 16 weeks, and then treated with a dose of 20 mg pure oleuropein daily for further 16 weeks, normalization of the blood glucose was observed.

The effect of the daily intake of 20 mg pure oleuropein in alloxan induced diabetic rabbits on lipid profile, uric acid, glycated hemoglobin, erythrocyte enzymatic antioxidant activity Superoxide dismutase (SOD), Glutathione reductase (GRx), Glutathione peroxidase (GPx), Glucose-6-phosphodehydrogenase (G-6PD), and glutathione (GSH) content, as well as non enzymatic antioxidant levels (vitamin C, vitamin E and β-carotene) in addition to parameters of oxidative stress, thiobarbituric acid reactant substances, and total antioxidant capacity were carried out in two parallel routes: alloxan induced diabetic rabbits administrated 20 mg of oleuropein daily for 16 weeks period and NIDDM patients administrated 1.0 gm of oleuropein daily for 6 months period. Significant changes in all parameters were observed.

Binding of I-^{125} insulin to intact human lymphocytes isolated from non insulin dependent diabetes mellitus patients was studied. The binding characteristics were studied and analyzed by scatchard plot. There was a high order low capacity binding sites with an affinity constant of 2×10^9 M^{-1} and a low order, high capacity binding sties with an affinity constant of 1.4×10^9 M^{-1}. The number of binding sites was significantly reduced in non-insulin dependent diabetes mellitus patients against healthy subjects. Long term administration of 1.0 gm of pure oleuropein daily for 6 months was associated with improvement in binding percent, protected the insulin receptors from oxidative damage, maintaining its functional integrity, and increase in both order of binding sites although no significant change in affinity constant was observed.

Finally the present study investigated for the first time the effect of oleuropein on histological changes possibly occurring in islets of Langerhans in pancreatic alloxan induced diabetic mice. Islets of Langerhans showed continuous hypertrophy with hyperplasia, lymphocyte infiltration and a significant increase in the average of islets diameter, while treatment with pure oleuropein showed a decrease average islet diameter with few small islets were atrophoid as a result of oleuropein intake, all of islets appeared normal as of the control animals.

1.1. Introduction

Natural compounds have been promising for medical potential, and some of these compounds stimulate the production of anti-cancer enzymes in the body. Others have antioxidant effects, protecting the body from oxidation damage caused by harmful molecular fragments known as free radicals that contribute to aging and illness. These natural compounds which called phytochemicals are found abundantly in roots, stems, leaves, fruits. They go by a variety of scientific names like polyphenols, secoiridoids, flavonoids, flavonols, isoprenoids, carotenoids, tocotrienols and proanthocyanadins [1].

Among the phytochemicals that have interest is oleuropein a substance found in the olive leaf, olive oil and olive fruit, a bitter principle of the leaves which was identified as oleuropeoside later designated oleuropein a polyphenolic secoiridoid glucoside by Panizzi [2] to which earlier reports of the hypotensive activity of the leaf extracts was accredited by Esdorn [3] and Stegmann [4]. Early experimental and clinical studies reported on the hypotensive effect of olive leaf extracted by different solvents and methods [5-6].

In 1991, Zarzuelo further investigated the hypotensive effect of a lypholized decoction of olive leaf and found it to be hypotensive and vasodilator on isolated aortae, the vasodilator effect being endothelium independent [7]. Others, however have shown that oleuropein increase nitric oxide synthase activity and the effect is blocked by N-nitro-L-arginine methyl ester [8].

Petkov and Manolov demonstrated the hypotensive as well as coronary vasodilator and anti-arrhythmic properties of oleuropein [9]. Olive leaf extracts have been employed experimentally to lower elevated blood-sugar levels in diabetic animals.Unfortunately, these results have not been reproduced in human clinical trials and as such, no clear conclusions can be made from this animal study in the treatment of diabetes [10].

Oleuropein is metabolized in the body to calcium elenolate, which is apparently responsible for many of the pharmacological actions of the olive leaf. Oleuropein is a heterosidic ester of elenolic acid and hydroxytyrosol, containing a molecule of glucose, the hydrolysis of which yields elenolic acid glucoside and hydroxytyrosol [11]. In vitro studies, it was demonstrated that oleuropein has the ability to inhibit proxidative processes on human low density lipoproteins [12]. Moreover, in vivo studies on rabbits have revealed that extra virgin olive oil biophenols, in particular oleuropein and hydroxytyrosol, are effective in preventing oxidation. In fact, supplementation of the diet with oleuropein decreased susceptibility to low density lipoprotein peroxidation and reduced the plasmatic levels of total, free, and ester cholesterol [12]. Many studies, carried out both *in vitro* and *in vivo*, have indicated that hydroxytyrosol is able to reduce the amount of isoprostane excreted in urine and hydroxytyrsol possesses strong antioxidant-scavenging ability contributing to the prevention of cardiovascular diseases, although *in vivo* studies have been performed to verify the antioxidant efficiency of oleuropein [13].

The reported findings on the hypoglycemic effects of olive leaf extract were not always consistent, possibly due to the instability of the extract and lack of proper standardization of its constituents. The iridoid glucoside of *olea europaea* leaves in particular easily undergoes rapid degradation if proper harvesting and extraction technologies are not implemented. Crude oleuropein, the main Iridoid glucoside in *olea europaea* leaf extract was shown to be degraded rapidly in aqueous solution but it remains stable in the pure form [14]. This made it necessary to test the activity of stabilized pure extract on one of the acknowledged models of experimental diabetes namely that by alloxan. Because of the paucity of literature concerning the effect of olive leaf extract as pure oleuropein on diabetic animals, it was decided to carry out the present investigation with oleuropein using model involved the use of rabbits rendered hyperglycemia by the administration of alloxan, as well as using human with non insulin dependent diabetes mellitus (NIDDM) as volunteers to carry out this study.

1.2. Literature   Review

1.2.1. *Olea europaea* L.

The olive tree, botanically-classified as *Olea europaea L.* is one of the most important fruit trees in Mediterranean countries. The characteristic green to blue-black fruit of this shrub yields useful edible oil. Both the oil and the dried green-grayish colored leaves are used medicinally [15].

The olive tree has been held in high esteem throughout history. The oil is symbolic of purity and goodness, while the olive branch represents peace and prosperity. Historically, the knowledge of the medicinal properties of the olive tree date back to the early 1800s, when it was used in liquid form for malaria treatment. In the early 1900s a bitter compound was found in the leaves of certain olive trees called "oleuropein," which was thought to be part of olive tree's potent disease-resistant structure [16].

The olive tree has been the source of natural healing agents down through the ages including the olive oil produced from its fruit. For centuries, teas and other preparations made from olive leaves have been used successfully to treat fevers and gastrointestinal complaints, including parasites in human patients. Olive leaf extract is effective against a broad spectrum of microbial agents, including viruses, bacteria and even parasites, and can considered one of the most useful and safe natural anti- microbial herbal extracts yet discovered [16-17]. It can inhibit and kill over 100 microorganisms which can cause disease and death on a broad scale, thus it can be considered nature antibiotic remedy to be used to prevent and treat numerous animal infectious conditions and health problems related to: viruses, bacteria, parasites, allergy conditions, skin problems (psoriasis), inflammation (arthritis, sinusitis, bursitis, etc.), gastrointestinal problems, ulcers, free radical overload, overburdened immune system, and wound healing [18-19].

The potent healing properties of olive leaf extracts in so many diverse areas make it one of the most comprehensive and versatile phytonutrients in products discovered to date. The principal active component in olive leaf extract is oleuropein, a natural product of the secoiridoid group. Upon hydrolysis, oleuropein can produce other bioactive fractions including elenolic acid. Oleuropein can be found in the olive trees bark, leaves, roots, wood and fruit where it protects the plant from nearly every insect and bacterial invader known and provides mankind with a truly remarkable therapeutic agent with broad health applications [20]. The olive tree has been called the Tree of Life [16]. With the revelation of the many wonderful healing properties of olive leaf extract now being clinically documented, this statement takes on a whole new meaning.

1.2.2. Olive leaf extract

The original olive leaf extract, as the name implies, derived from the leaves of the olive tree. It is a source of many phytochemicals [2]. It was found to be part of a compound produced by olive trees that make them particularly vigorous and resistant to insect and bacterial damage [17] The *Olea europaea* L. leaves represent a typical herbal drug of the Mediterranean area, commonly used in traditional medicine as vasodilatory, hypotensive, anti-inflammatory, antirheumatic, diuretic' antipyretic, and hypoglycemic agents [21-27].

The active constituents of olive leaf have a wide number of ingredients, including the chief constituent oleuropein (60-90 mg/g) and several types of polyphenolic compounds. The following polyphenols were detected in olive leaf tissue: hydroxytyrosol, hydroxytyrosol glucoside, tyrosol, elenolic acid derivatives, caffeic acid, oleuropein, verbascoside, rutin, luteolin 7-O-glucoside, luteolin 4-O-glucoside, apigenin-7-O-rutinoside and apigenin 7-O-glucoside [28-29]. There are at least six active substances (oleuropein, hydroxytyrosol, caffeic acid, vanillin, luteolin-7-glucoside, and verbascoside) in the extract. These six substances work together synergistically to prevent resistance by pathogen microorganisms. While oleuropein is the ingredient most studied, there are in fact 95 different chemicals in the leaf and a balance of ingredients seems to work the best. Oleuropein content varies from 17% to 23% depending upon the time of year the leaves are harvested [30].

1.2.3. Pharmacologic effects of olive leaf extracts

1.2.3.1. *Antimicrobial effect*

Olive leaf extract has been used as a natural antibiotic for thousands of years, but it is only recently that scientific research has shown that its active ingredient oleuropein, has powerful healing properties, and can fight bacteria, viruses, fungi and parasites that cause infections and disease[18,19,20]. Oleuropein possesses direct anti-viral, anti-bacterial and anti-parasitic activity when taken orally or applied topically. Antimicrobial activity occurs in the body when **d-** Elenolic is used because oleuropein breaks down to elenolic acid (in the form of calcium elenolate; a calcium salt [16]. Elenolic acid interacts with a target pathogen at a receptor, in the same way a key interacts with a lock. The Elenolic acid is the key and the pathogen receptor is the lock. Left-handed Elenolic acid binds completely (100%) to serum protein, which prevents interaction with pathogen receptors while right-handed Elenolic acid (key) fits the pathogen receptor (lock), the pathogen is inhibited or destroyed [31].

Oleuropein breaks down in the body to produce Elenolic acid, a compound which has shown exceptional virucidal and bactericidal activity against all viruses and bacteria for which it has been tested [17-18]. Oleuropein is able to enhance the immune response and enable the body to fight infection more effectively. There are specific ways that oleuropein is able to work against microbes. They include:

- Interfering with certain amino acid production processes necessary to keep the pathogen alive.
- Inactivating viruses by interfering with virus shedding, budding or assembly at the cellular membrane.
- Neutralizing retrovirus by preventing production of the viral enzymes, reverse transcriptase and protease needed by the retrovirus to alter the RNA of a healthy cell. This is true for the human immunodeficiency virus (HIV).
- Stimulating phagocytosis, immune system response in which macrophages ingest microorganisms and foreign substances.

Oleuropein, via its breakdown into elenolic acid within the cell is able to directly penetrate infected host cells and irreversibly inhibit viral replication. It also works on latent viruses as well apparently without influencing other mechanisms or reactions of the host cell. This remarkable property may explain why is completely nontoxic. Olive leaf extract is recommended for colds, cold sores (herpes,) flu, ear infections, eye infections, nose and throat infections, impetigo, pink eye, parasites, and most bacterial, viral and fungal infections., AIDS, herpes, Epstein-Barr, bladder infections, skin infections, eczema, fungus and yeast infections, malaria and surprisingly, psoriasis, hemorrhoids, arrhythmias, and rheumatoid arthritis. There is a theory, that rheumatoid arthritis may be caused by infectious agents (such as mycoplasma) and it would be interesting to try it against other diseases that are suspected to be caused by infectious agents such as multiple sclerosis. [1, 32]

Olive leaf extract as a therapeutic agent, goes beyond its antimicrobial activity. Research shows it also has antioxidant and anti-inflammatory properties which are especially beneficial for aiding cardiovascular disease, yeast infections and inflammatory conditions [1, 33].

1.2.3.2. *Cardiovascular effect*

Olive leaf extract is beneficial for both coronary heart disease (CHD) and peripheral vascular disease (PVD).Visioli F, et al reported that oleuropein protects, as an antioxidant, low density lipoproteins from oxidation and interferes with the biochemical events that lead to atherosclerosis[8]. Oleuropein has similar antioxidant properties of various polyphenolic compounds and flavonoids that protect the cardiovascular system. Esdom has reported that olive leaf extract is effective in reducing hypertension and can help eliminate arterial fibrillation which usually leads to the implantation of a permanent pace maker [3]. Arterial fibrillation is a heart condition marked by rapid, irregular heart rate from 130 to 150 beats per minute. Studies down by Circosta et al was reported a significant decrease in high blood pressure in patients after being on olive leaf extract for three months[6]. The investigators found that it reduced both systolic and diastolic blood pressures [14] .Multiple animal studies have confirmed olive leaf extracts ability to reduce hypertension as well to normalize arrhythmic action of the heart [3].

Olive leaf extract was found to inhibit oxidation of low-density lipoproteins, the so-called "bad cholesterol" involved in heart and arterial disease. This revelation, if confirmed by further research, suggests that oleuropein may contain antioxidant properties similar to other phytochemicals compounds [8, 9, and 34]. Studies have shown that some phytochemicals can reduce the harmful oxidation of cholesterol as well as slow down the accelerated clumping of blood platelets that can lead to dangerous clots [8]. Olive leaf extract was found to cause relaxation of arterial walls in laboratory animals. Such results suggest a possible benefit for hypertension, an effect first mentioned by researchers more than 30 years ago [7, 35]. The aqueous extract of olive leaves was found to reduce hypertension, blood sugar, and the level of uric acid in rodents[26,27].. These findings again indicate potential in the treatment of hypertension, as well as diabetes and heart disease [34]. Specific areas where olive leaf extract is effective include: atherosclerosis, arterial fibrillation, angina pectoris, arrhythmias intermittent claudication, impaired circulation and hypertension [7, 35].

1.2.3.3. *Anti-parasite effect*

Parasites are notoriously difficult to kill and expel from the body. Olive leaf extract exhibits powerful anti-parasitic action against just such invaders. Olive leaf extract may offer considerable potential in the treatment of tropical infections such as malaria and dengue. As far back as 1827, reports have appeared in medical literature indicating the benefits of olive leaf extract in the treatment of malaria. In 1906 one report stated that olive leaves were, in fact, superior to quinine for malarial infections. Quinine was preferred, however, because it was easier to administer. Recently many studies reported that calcium elenolate, the substance within oleuropein, was found to be effective against the malaria protozoa [17].

1.2.3.4. *Anti-inflammatory effect*

As mentioned earlier, olive leaf extract also is a potent anti-inflammatory preparation which can be very effective against a number of inflammatory conditions caused by: degenerative joint disease, bursitis, sinusitis, wounds and skin conditions like psoriasis. Oleuropein is the apparent active anti-inflammatory factor in olive leaf extract although there may be other anti-inflammatory flavonoids present as well. Olive leaves extract work well to bring relief of the pain and swelling associated with the above conditions [36, 39].

1.2.3.5. *Immune- stimulant effect*

Olive leaf extract empowers the immune system by directly stimulating production of the immune system cells called phagocytes. These phagocytes move throughout the body looking for foreign invaders. They then neutralize any abnormal organisms that they find. An important fact is that microbes cannot be resistant to phagocyte cells like they can to drug interventions. Olive leaf extract contains flavonoids, esters and multiple iridoids that create a structurally-complicated molecule [1]. It appears that bad microorganisms cannot readily develop a resistance to olive leaf extract's complex structure. Olive leaf extract does not disturb the beneficial bacteria in the intestines. Already olive leaf extract has shown itself to be the only effective and nutritional remedy available for the fatal Bacillus cereus contamination. This is a microorganism that infects the body and there is no known medical treatment or cure once infected, it takes over the body and the person dies. Tassou et al investigated that olive leaf extract and oleuropein inhibit the germination and growth of the pathogen. [20]

1.2.3.6. *Toxological effect*

The only adverse effect of using olive leaf extract to fight off an active infection is a counter response known as the Herxheimer reaction. It is caused by a large "die-off of the pathological organism causing the infection, which in turn may lead to an allergic or toxic overload effect. The body's own immune system destroys the dead bacteria and the breakdown products can cause a variety of toxic symptoms[1].. Some detoxification symptoms may occur with the initial use of olive leaf extract as it kills bad microbes faster than the body can eliminate them. This is easily remedied by reducing the dosage for a few days to allow the animal's waste disposal system to catch up. Once the cleaning takes place, which may take up to several days. Energy levels will increase and the symptoms will subside [32].

1.2.4. Oleuropein

The secoiridoid oleuropein is the bitter principle of olives and is found in olive oil as such and in its aglycone form. It was first named and studied by Bourquelot [38] and investigated in humans by Panizzi who reported on the hypotensive properties of this complex phenol [2]. Oleuropein is a heterosidic ester of elenolic acid and 3, 4-dihydroxy-phenylethanol (hydroxytyrosol), containing a molecule of glucose, the hydrolysis of which yields elenolic acid glucoside and hydroxytyrosol (Fig.1-1).Oleuropein is metabolized to calcium elenolate when is taken orally by two natural enzymes in the body esterase and beta-glucosidase [31].This elenolic acid is apparently responsible for many of the pharmacological actions of the olive leaf extract [11]. Oleuropein is a phenolic secoiridoid glucoside widespread in members of the family

Oleaceae. It has been shown to possess a wide range of biological activities. It increased coronary blood flow and showed anti- arrhythmic and spasmolytic effects [9, 14].

Oleuropein exhibited hypoglycemic effect and increased tolerance of orally administered glucose [26-27]. It also showed anti-oxidative and anti-inflammatory properties [8]. Other reported effects of oleuropein included the potentiation of cellular and organism protection through the macrophage-mediated response, the inhibition of platelet aggregation and eicosanoid production [39], reduction of the low density lipoprotcins (LDL) level, potent and protective antioxidant action on LDL,[12] inhibitory effects on cytochrome P450 and 17-β-hydroxysteroid dehydrogenase activity, Potent toxic effects on tumor cell lines, and antibacterial functions. Recently, oleuropein was also claimed in a U.S. patent to have potent antiviral activities against herpes mononucleosis, hepatitis virus, rotavirus, bovine rhinovirus, canine parvovirus and feline leukemia virus [36,40].

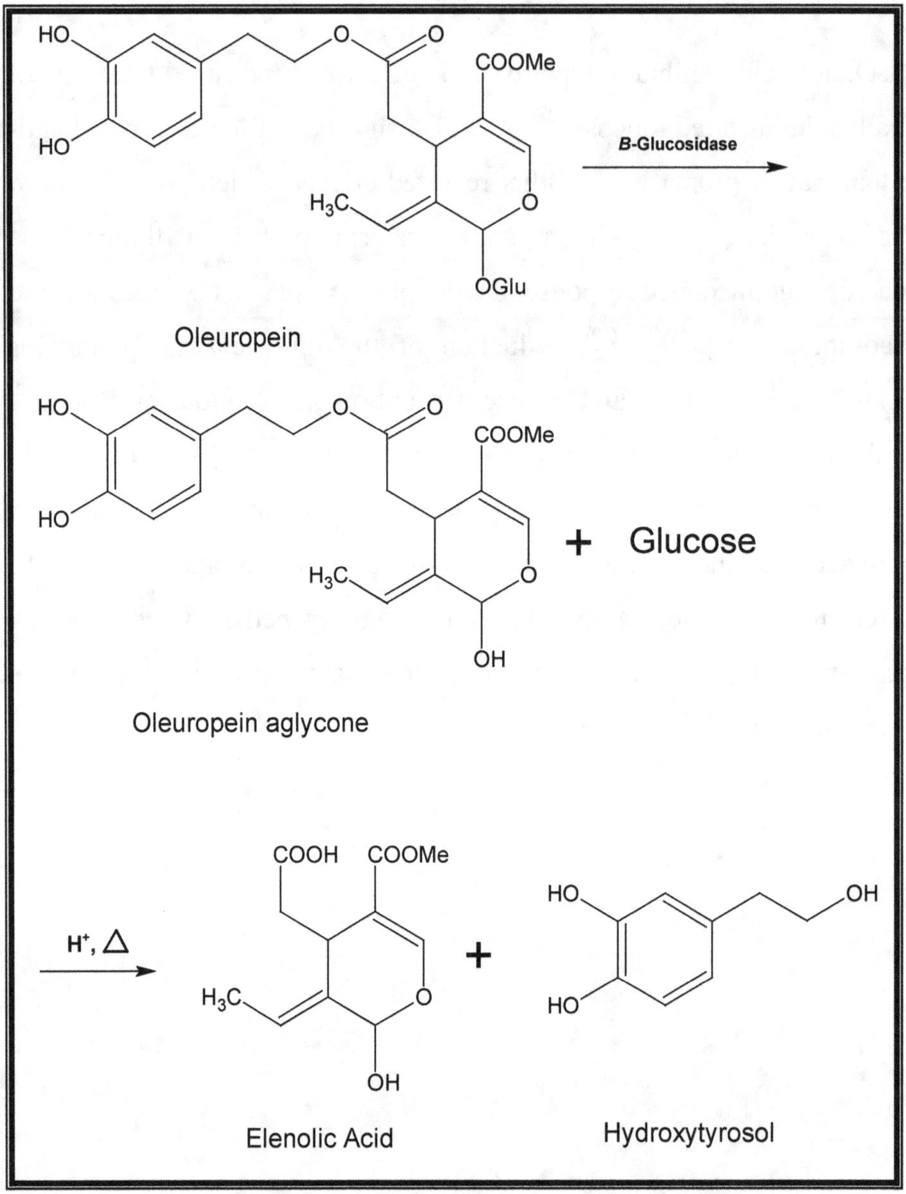

Figure 1-1. The degradation products of enzymatic and acidic hydrolysis of oleuropein [31]

1.2.4.1. Distribution of oleuropein in olives

1.2.4.1.1. *Oleuropein content in olive leaf*

The amount of oleuropein in olive leaves depends on several factors, including *olea europeae* variety (olives from the Coratina variety are the richest in phenolic compounds especially oleuropein), time of collection , possible infestation by the olive fly Dacus Olea, climate, conditions of storage, and the methodology of extraction [41-43]. Oleuropein content varies from 17% to 23% depending upon the time of year the leaves are harvested [30]. By using a mixture of methanol/water a best recovery of R-oleuropein reached 30% of the extract can be obtained [42, 44].

1.2.4.1.2. *Oleuropein content in olive fruit*

The contents of oleuropein in olives vary widely according to the literature. Variations in the content of phenolic compounds within one species is mainly due to differences in the olive varieties or in growth conditions, type of irrigation used and also methodological differences may contribute to the variability in the reported oleuropein concentrations. Discrepancies found may be also partly being due to differences in the maturity stage of the fruits [43-44]. Accumulation of oleuropein varies strongly in relation to the physiological state of the fruit, leaves, being a result of equilibrium between biosynthesis and further metabolism including turnover and catabolism. The most important control mechanisms in the phenolic metabolism include the amount of enzymes, regulation of enzyme activities, compartmentation of enzymes, availability of precursors and intermediates, and integration in the differentiation and development programs [45].

Numerous investigations have confirmed that concentrations of phenolic compounds (oleuropein) are higher in young fruits. Oleuropein amounts to up to 14% of the dry weight in unripe olives, but during maturation, undergoes hydrolysis and yields several simpler molecules that build up the well known olive oil complex taste. Oleuropein is the major ortho-diphenolic in olive fruit. Concentrations of this compound vary considerably both during life of the fruit and according to the cultivar, green or black, table of pressing [44-45].

Browning capacity of olive fruits come from complex interactions between diphenol oxidase activity and oleuropein content. There is a positive correlation between browning and oleuropein content. Oleuropein content was high in young fruits, falls considerably at the beginning of the green maturation and then stabilized. Elenolic acid glucoside and hydroxytyrosol are indicators of the maturation of olives since they increase as the fruit ripens, whereas the amount of the OLE decreases. This could be correlated to the increase activity of the hydrolytic enzymes [44]. In particular, glucosidase catalyze the hydrolysis of the OLE with the production of OLE aglycone and the dialdehyde form of elenolic acid linked to hydroxytyrosol [45-47]. Oleuropein is always present, even in the 1-year aged samples stored at 5-10 C°, and its content ranges up to the interesting value of 11.3% (w/w) which as previously mentioned [46].

1.2.4.1.3. *Oleuropein content in olive oil*

Since the oleuropein content of virgin olive oil is influenced by the variety of *olea europeae,* location, degree of ripeness and the type of oil extraction process used [42]. Oleuropein in olive oil amount to up 500mg/kg although, due to the variety of methods proposed for their determination, the reported values are hardly comparable. The widely employed Folin-Ciocalteau reagent is not specific for phenols and HPLC procedures are limited by the complexity of the phenolic fraction. The absolute concentration of phenolic compounds in olive oil is the result of a complex interaction between several factors, including cultivar, degree of maturation and climate it usually decreases with over-maturation of olives, although there are some exceptions to this rule .For instance, olive grown in warmer climates, despite a more rapid maturation, yield oils that are rich in phenols. It is noteworthy that during the elaboration of olive oil, a considerable amounts of phenols, according to their partition coefficient; end up in the wastewater [48].

1.2.4.2. Antioxidant activities of oleuropein

1.2.4.2.1. *In vitro studies*

The epidemiological evidence of a lower incidence of coronary heart disease (CHD) in the Mediterranean area led to the hypothesis of a protective effect of some olive oil phenolic, with respect to chemically induced oxidation of human LDL, i.e., one of the key steps in the initiation of atherosclerosis [49-50]. The recent availability of pure compounds, namely hydroxytyrosol and, oleuropein, stimulated research in this field. Oxidation of LDL can be investigated in vitro by incubating isolated LDL with a variety of oxidative agents, including chemicals such as transition metal ions and azo-compounds, cultured cells such as macrophages and endothelial cells, or by physical means such as UV light radiation [51]. Several markers of oxidative stress must be taken into account, as they provide information on the oxidative modifications of lipids and apolipoproteins [51].

Both hydroxytyrosol and oleuropein potently inhibit copper sulfate-induced oxidation of LDL in a dose-dependent manner, at concentrations of 20 μM [8, 51]. The protective effects of hydroxytyrosol and oleuropein are demonstrated through the assessment of various markers, such as a reduced formation of short-chain aldehydes and of lipid peroxides, by higher vitamin E content in the residual LDL and by a reduced formation of malondialdehyde-lysine and 4-hydroxynonenal-lysine adducts, indicating protection of the apoprotein layer. The antioxidant activities of hydroxytyrosol and oleuropein, which have been proven to be more effective than beta-hydroxytolune (BHT) or vitamin E, were further confirmed, by the use of metal- independent oxidative systems [52] and stable free radicals, such as 2,2-diphenyl-1-picrylhydrazyl (DPPH) in a series of experiments that demonstrated both a strong metal-chelation and a free-radical scavenging action[11]. In particular, both hydroxytyrosol and oleuropein scavenged superoxide anions generated by either human polymorph nuclear cells or by the xanthine/xanthine oxidase system. Furthermore, a scavenging effect of hydroxytyrosol and oleuropein were demonstrated with respect to hypochlorous acid, a potent oxidant produced *in vivo* at the site of inflammation [53-54].

In fact, although specific investigations on the structure-activity relationship of olive oil phenols are yet to be carried out, similar studies have been performed on flavonoids and have indicated that the degree of antioxidant activity is correlated with the number of hydroxyl substitutions [55]. Particularly, the ortho-dihydroxy substitution confers a high antioxidant capacity, whereas single hydroxyl substitutions, as in the case of tyrosol, provide no activity. The activities of hydroxytyrosol toward chemically-induced DNA and amino acid modifications have been investigated by some researchers [52, 56].

1.2.4.2.2. *Effect of oleuropein on enzymes activity*

Olive oil phenolics are amphiphilic and they partition between the lipid (oil) and water (waste water) phases; their activities on enzymes potentially sensitive to phenolic compounds were tested in a variety of cellular models, i.e., platelets, leukocytes, macrophages. Indeed, lipid-soluble antioxidants such as tocopherols are unable to affect enzymes such as cyclo- and lipoxygenases, NAD(P)H oxidase, and nitric oxide synthase that are involved in key functions of those cells. Hydroxytyrosol has been therefore tested for activities in addition to its antioxidant properties, such as the in vitro effect on platelet function, where the compound was proven to inhibit the chemically induced aggregation, the accumulation of the pro-aggregant agent thromboxane in human serum, the production of the pro-inflammatory molecules leukotrienes by activated human leukocytes, and the inhibition of arachidonate lipoxygenase [8, 57, 58]. For instance, when added to murine macrophages together with a bacterial lipopolysaccharide, oleuropein increases the functional activity of these immune competent cells, as evaluated by a significant increase ($58.7 \pm 4.6\%$) in the production of the bactericidal and cytostatic factor nitric oxide [11, 58]. This increase was due to a direct tonic effect of oleuropein on the inducible form of the enzyme nitric oxide synthase (iNOS), as demonstrated by Western blot analysis of cell sonicates and by the co-incubation of LPS-challenged cells with the iNOS inhibitor L-nitromethylarginine methyl ester. Finally, macrophage nitric oxide exerts a protective role in preventing oxidative LDL modification [8].

The hypothesis was tested that both oleuropein and hydroxytyrosol possess estrogenic or androgenic activities [59]. The potency of olive phenols as antioxidants suggests that they could be fruitfully employed as prophylactic agents; this might be particularly true in the case of olive mill waste waters, from where highly purified extracts that contain a high proportion of hydroxytyrosol can be obtained [59].

1.2.4.2.3. *In vivo studies*

In addition to the large body of epidemiological data, experimental evidence that phenolic compounds are uptaken from the diet is accumulating. Experiments with laboratory animals, for example rats or rabbits, have demonstrated a higher resistance to oxidation of LDL obtained from animals fed virgin olive oil, as compared to animals that were only given a triglyceride preparation with an equivalent amount of oleic acid, i.e., triolein [60] "plain" olive oil [61].

Visioli et al demonstrated that olive oil phenolic are dose-dependently absorbed in humans and that they are excreted in the urine as glucuronide conjugates[53] interestingly, increasing amounts of phenolic administered with olive oil stimulated the rate of conjugation with glucuronic acid. Finally, the postprandial absorption of olive oil phenolic and their incorporation into human lipoproteins has been reported by Bonanome [62,]. These data add to the experimental evidence indicating absorption and disposition of some flavonoids in humans [63-65]. It is worth speculating that the low bioavailability at times attributed to various phenols and flavonoids such as quercetin, luteolin, and apigenin after ingestion of diverse plant foods [63-64] might be attributed to their strong interactions with the food matrix, as in the case with artichokes, carrots, etc. This is not the case of olive oil phenolics, which are easily transferred to the oil by the pressing of the drupe and then are simply dissolved in olive oil. Also, a low dose of hydroxytyrosol ($414\mu g$/rat) was able to inhibit passive smoking-induced oxidative stress in rats, as demonstrated by a reduced urinary excretion of the F2–isoprostane (8-iso-PGF$_{2a}$) [65].

Finally, a dose-dependent inverse correlation between the rate of 8-iso-PGF$_{2a}$ excretion and increasing amounts of phenolic ingested with olive oil was observed in human volunteers, interestingly, the urinary levels of 8-iso-PGF$_{2a}$ inversely correlated with those of homovanillyl alcohol, i.e., a catechol-O-methyl-transferase (COMT)-derived metabolite of hydroxytyrosol. Manna et al. (1999) suggested that the latter enters into cellular compartments where it exerts its antioxidant activity [66].

1.2.4.3. *Bioavailability of oleuropein*

Oleuropein is a heterosidic ester of elenolic acid and hydroxytyrosol containing a molecule of glucose, the hydrolysis of which yields elenolic acid glucoside and hydroxytyrosol [13]. Although *in vivo* studies have been performed to verify the antioxidant efficiency of oleuropein, reports of its bioavailability and biological fate are very scare and data indicating the circulating concentration of oleuropein and its bioactive metabolites after oral administration are absent. Hydroxytyrosol and oleuropein are the most representative catecholic components of olives and their derivatives, including extra virgin olive oil, olive leaf extract and olive mill waste water [11, 67]. Hydroxytyrosol is also a constituent of the OLE moiety, which is normally found in olive leaf and oil in its aglycone form (OLEa), and represents the bioactive portion of the OLE molecule [68]. In vitro, both compounds exhibit potent antioxidant and enzyme-modulating activities [65, 69].

Recently, several in vivo studies [12,62,65,70-72] proved that olive oil phenolic are dose-dependently absorbed after oral administration to rats and humans, in which they are metabolized and excreted in the urine mostly as glucuronide conjugates (Figure 1-2). Published data show that hydroxytyrosol retains its antioxidant activities following ingestion [73]. Analytical methods suitable for the measurement of oleuropein and hydroxytyrosol from biological tissues are mainly based on HPLC and GC-MS, the latter being used particularly for hydroxytyrosol [74]. Recently, several studies have measured the level of hydroxytyrosol in human plasma using an HPLC- UV system and in rat plasma either by LC-MS or GC-MS analysis. More recently, Vissers M., described the absorption of olive oil hydroxyl phenols in humans by measuring oleuropein and hydroxytyrosol by HPLC and GC-MS, respectively [70-76].

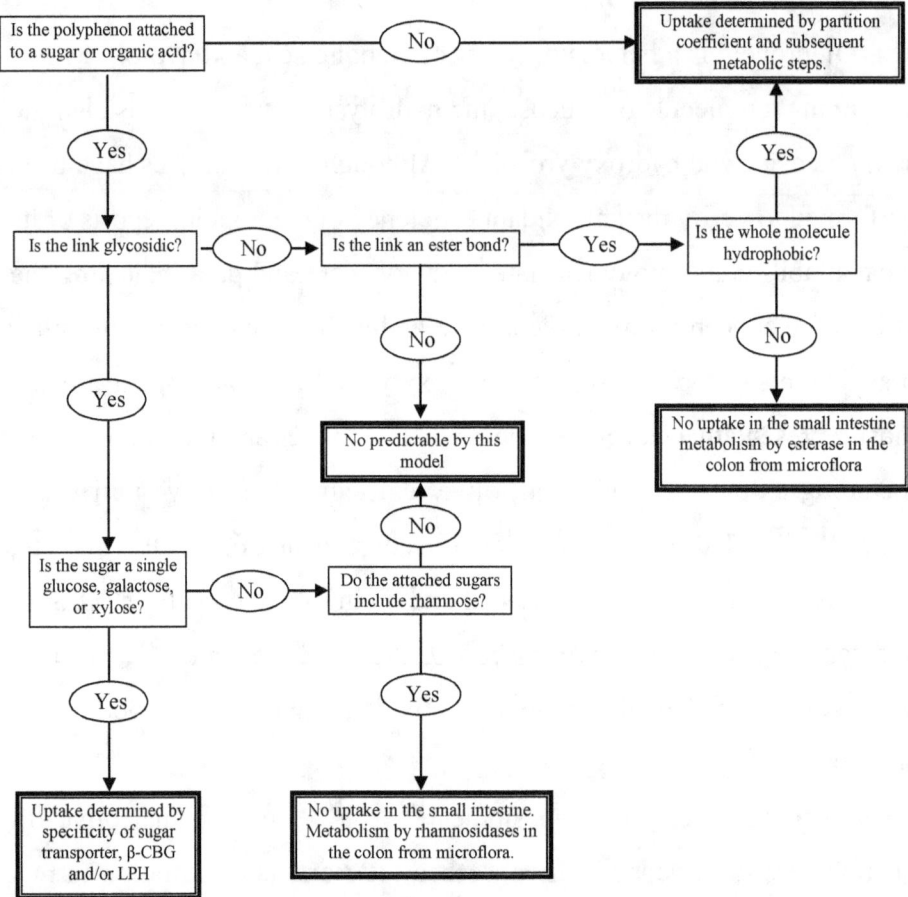

Figure 1-2. Hypothesis for prediction of the absorption of polyphenols in humans based on evidence from in vivo and in vitro studies. [76]

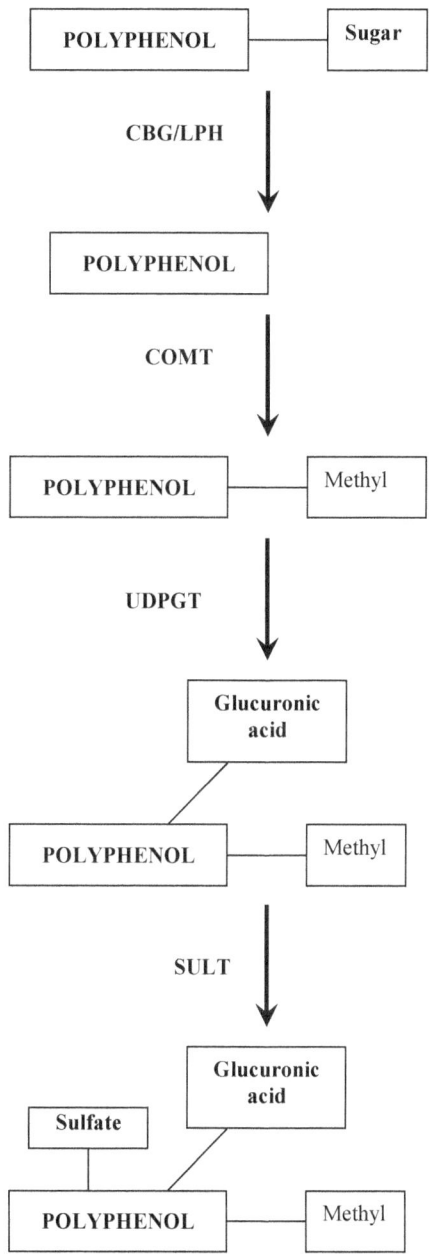

Figure 1-3. Simplified scheme showing the metabolism of polyphenols [76]

To better characterize the precise pharmacokinetic properties of oleuropein, it is important to develop a highly sensitive and simple analytical method for its quantization in biological samples. Therefore, an accurate LC-MS/MS methodology for the simultaneous detection of oleuropein and hydroxytyrosol in rat plasma and urine following oral ingestion of oleuropein was developed and this method was validated and applied *in vivo* [75].

Oleuropein was determined in plasma, and then metabolized to hydroxytyrosol as the major product, and as glucuronide derivatives in urine (Figure 1-3, 1-4). These results demonstrate that oleuropein is absorbed and converted enzymatically into hydroxytyrosol, the latter having relevant antioxidant properties. Piero Del B., (2003) described a new LC-MS method for the simultaneous measurement of oleuropein and hydroxytyrosol in rat plasma and urine [75].

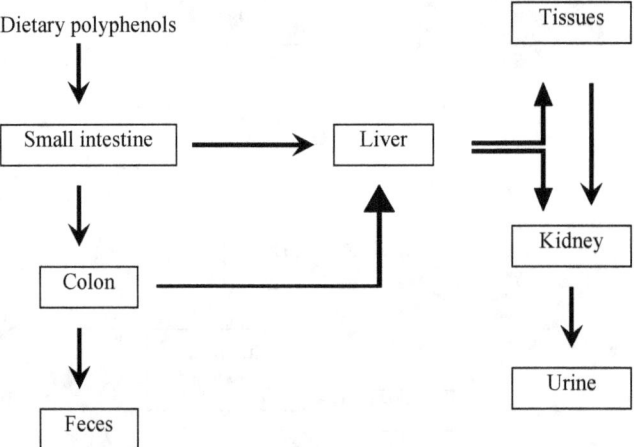

Figure 1-4. Possible routes for consumed polyphenols in humans
(76)

It appears that oleuropein is absorbed after oral administration, since it was found in plasma and in urine, and hydroxytyrosol was its most relevant metabolite. Oleuropein and hydroxytyrosol could be quantified as low as 2.5 and 5 ng /ml in plasma and urine, respectively. Moreover, it appears that oleuropein is absorbed rapidly considering the maximum of 2 hours [65].

Oleuropein and hydroxytyrosol were recovered in urine mainly as glucuronide, and in very low concentrations as free forms. This is due to the instability of these free forms in urine, as demonstrated. In plasma samples, oleuropein was present only as the glucoside, whereas hydroxytyrosol was found only in traces as the free form. The simultaneous quantification method using LC- MS is specific, sensitive and accurate for the determination of these important dietary components and for investigating their bioavailability and metabolism, in view of their consideration as potential therapeutic agents [75].

1.2.5. Analytical methods

1.2.5.1. *Extraction and hydrolysis techniques of phenolic acids*

The most common solvents used for the extraction of phenolic acids from plant matrices are ethyl acetate [77], diethyl ether [78-79], methanol or aqueous methanol [80]. Enzymatic hydrolysis with β-glucosidase [81] or hydrocinnamoyl-quinate esterase has been applied for the analysis of phenolic acids [82].

Acid hydrolysis has been done by heating the sample with HC1 for 2 hours or more [83-84]. Hydrolysis of benzoic acid and cinnamic acid esters with alkali can be performed with NaOH at room temperature for 4-24 hours or for 90 min at 60 °C [84].

Rommel and Wrolstad (1993a) tested acid (HC1) and base (NaOH) hydrolysis in the analysis of phenolic composition (ellagic acid, hydroxybenzoic acids, hydroxycinnamic acids, flavonols and flavan-3-ols) of olive fruit [85].

The phenolic pattern of the alkaline hydrolyzed sample was very similar to that of the acid hydrolyzed sample of the same fruit. Only one ellagic acid compound was hydrolyzed more effectively in alkaline than in acidic conditions. In general, optimization of extraction and hydrolysis conditions is always needed when phenolic acids are quantified from fruits or leaves or other plant materials [83].

1.2.6.2. *Chromatographic techniques*

Paper chromatographic methods were developed for flavonoids in the 1950s and 1960s [86] .These techniques were replaced by thin layer chromatography (TLC) in the 1970s providing an inexpensive and useful technique for the simultaneous analysis of several samples [77]. Selection of a suitable stationary phase and solvent depends on the classes of flavonoids to be examined. Hydrophilic flavonoids, such as flavonols, can be readily separated by TLC on polyamide or microcrystalline cellulose. TLC is still in common use for preparative separations [83], and as a rapid low cost screening method for determining the flavonoid classes present in fruits and leaves [79]. TLC applications for quantitative analysis of phenolic acids are usually carried out using normal phase chromatography on cellulose or silica layers and separating the compounds with a mixture of hydrocarbon carriers (toluene, dioxan or benzene) and polar organic modifiers (acetone, butanol, ethanol or acetic acid) [77].

The advantages in screening the sample extract by TLC prior to HPLC are the detection of contaminants that may absorb to the stationary phase in the HPLC column, or the determination of solvent conditions necessary for a successful separation of phenolic compounds. A TLC method was developed to detect major polyphenols in olive oil involving RP-TLC and silica gel high performance TLC [87].

Gas chromatography (GC) has only a limited applicability in the analysis of flavonoids and other phenolic due to their limited volatility; the main disadvantage is an extra step required to ensure the volatility of the phenolic. [83,86]. However, GC analysis with mass spectrometric (MS) detection has been applied for the analysis of flavonols in black tea [88]. Advantages of GC analysis include an improved separation of closely related isomers and simple coupling to MS detectors for identification through the fragmentation pattern [89-90]. A new gas chromatography method for determination the phenolic compounds in virgin olive oil was developed by Angerosa [91].

High-performance liquid chromatography (HPLC) has been the most widely employed chromatographic technique in flavonoid analysis during the past 20 years [86]. It has added a new dimension to the investigation of flavonoids in plant and food extracts. Particular advantages are the improved resolution of flavonoid mixtures compared to other chromatographic techniques, the ability to obtain both qualitative and accurate quantitative data in one operation, and the great speed of analysis [92].

Normal-phase chromatography has been used for the separation of flavonoids (flavone, flavonol and flavanone aglycone) in olive oil. Flavonoid acetates were separated isocratically on LiChrosorb Si60 using benzene-acetonitril, benzene-ethanol or iso-octane-ethanol-acetonitrile solvent systems and detected at 312 or 270 nm. However, for normal-phase systems, there is a concern that highly polar materials may be irreversibly retained in the column [93] with the result that the separation characteristics could be gradually altered. Thus, reversed-phase (RP) chromatography has invariably been the method of choice for the separation of flavonols, other flavonoid groups and phenolic compounds in olive fruit and leaves. The normal way of separation uses a C 18 column (particle size 3-5 μm) together with aqueous mobile phases and methanol or acetonitril as an organic modifier. Small amounts of acetic acid, formic acid or phosphate buffers incorporated in the mobile phase tend to markedly improve separations of flavonoids and other phenolic compounds [92].

The pH and ionic strength of the mobile phase are known to influence the retention of phenolic in the column depending on protonation, dissociation, or a partial dissociation [94]. A change in pH which increases the ionisation of a sample could reduce the retention in a reversed-phase separation. Thus, small amounts of acetic (2-5%), formic, phosphoric or trifluoroacetic acid (0.1%) are included in the solvent system to suppress ionisation of phenolic and carboxylic groups and hence to improve resolution and reproducibility of chromatographic runs [95].

1.2.6.3. *Detection and identification of flavonols and phenolic acids*

Phenolic compounds absorb in the UV region and the most commonly used detector for HPLC is a variable-wavelength UV or UV-visible detector [86]. No single wavelength is ideal for monitoring all classes of phenolic since they display absorbance maxima at different wavelengths [96]. Most benzoic acid derivatives display their maxima at 246-262 nm, except for gallic acid and syringic acid which have absorption maxima at 271 and 275 nm, respectively,[97] Hydroxycinnamic acids absorb in two UV regions, one maximum being in the range of 225-235 nm and the other in the range of 290-330 nm [98]. At 320 nm, cinnamic acid derivatives can be detected without any interference from benzoic acid derivatives, which have a higher absorptivity at 254 nm. However, detection at 280 nm is the best alternative for the determination of both classes of phenolic compounds [99].The absorption range 350-370 nm has been widely used for flavonol aglycone and 280 nm for flavan-3-ol and flavonol glycosides [86].

The extensive use of photo-diode array detection (PDA) in the analysis of flavonoids and phenolic acids can be attributed to the ability to collect on-line spectra [99] without using stopped-flow techniques. This has led to a considerable improvement in the HPLC analysis for identification purposes and demonstrated the usefulness of qualitative information in phenolic analysis that is based on the absorption spectrum [100]. PDA has three major advantages: multiple wavelength detection, peak identification, and peak purity determination [100]. The UV detection has the disadvantage of not being as sensitive or selective as fluorescence detection, and interfering peaks are more common. However, fluorescence detection has not been applied widely to phenolic [101]. In the analysis of phenolic in olive fruits, fluorescence detection offers major advantages over UV detection in terms of enhanced selectivity and sensitivity [101]. HPLC-MS is a fast and reliable method for structural analyses of non-volatile phenolic compounds, since better techniques have been developed for the removal of the liquid mobile phase before ionisation [102].

Pietta et al. (1994) showed that thermospray liquid chromatography LC- MS is an excellent technique for the analysis of flavonol glycosides from medicinal plants and various groups of polyphenols including flavonol glycosides in tea have been studied using thermospray LC-MS [103].

Positive ion fast atom bombardment MS and tandem MS have been used to study the glycosidic linkages in oleuropein [104,105] as shown in figure (1-12). Electrospray and its several variations are more recent developments in atmospheric pressure ionization mass spectrometers [102-103]. HPLC electrospray ionization (ESI)-MS offers advantages in terms of sensitivity and capacity for the analysis of large, thermally labile and highly polar compounds [102-103].

Ryan D. et al (1999) demonstrated the potential of electrospray ionization mass spectrometry for the specific detection of phenolic species in olives [101] as shown in figure (1-13) also; Enzo P et al. (1999) demonstrated the presence of oleuropein in virgin olive oil by ionspray tandem mass spectrometry (ISI-MS/MS) [106]. Atmospheric pressure ionization (API)-MS technique has been applied for the analysis of flavonoids and phenolic compounds in olive leaves. [107]

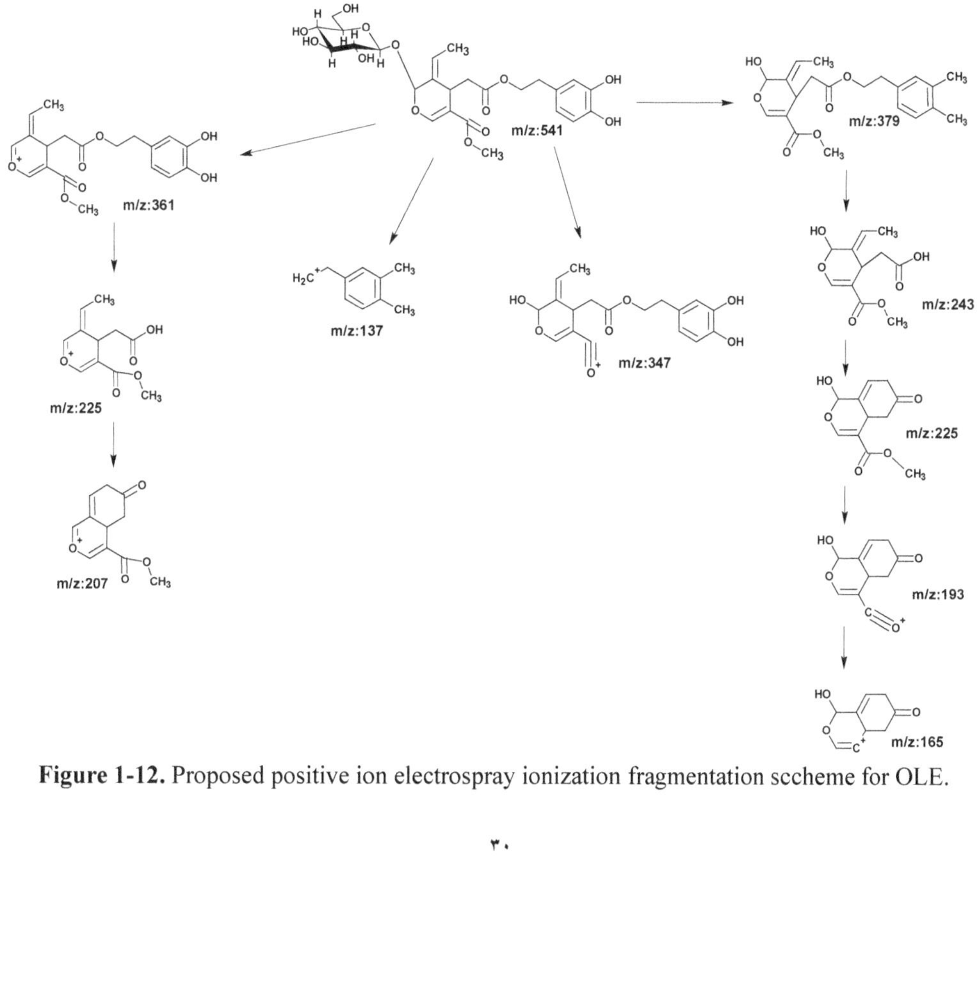

Figure 1-12. Proposed positive ion electrospray ionization fragmentation sccheme for OLE.

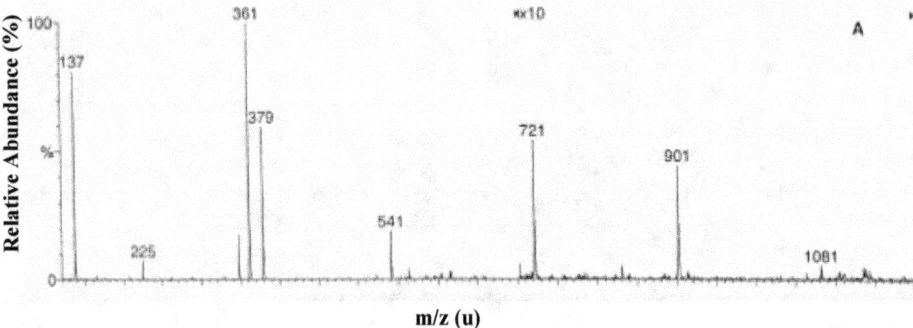

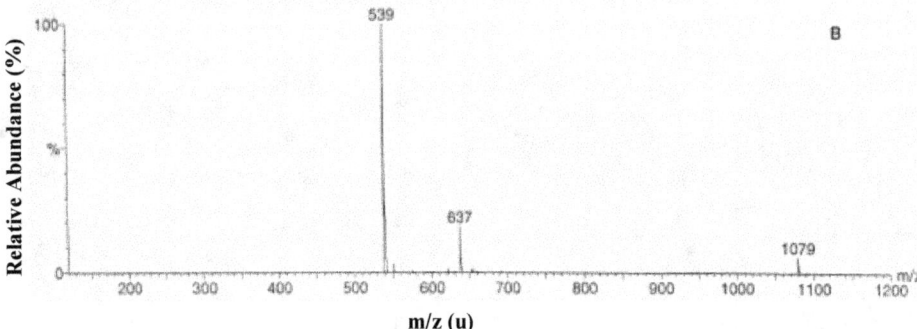

Figure 1-13. Mass spectrum of oleuropein by Electrospray ionisation method. (A) Positive ion mass spectrum. The region above *m/z* 700 is magnified 10 times. (B) Negative ion mass spectrum [107

1.2.7. Diabetes Mellitus

1.2.7.1. *Adverse effects of type 2 diabetes*

Type 2 diabetes as known non insulin dependent diabetes mellitus (NIDDM) is characterized by an increased risk for the development of macrovascular disease (coronary heart disease, cerebrovascular disease, and peripheral vascular disease) and microvascular complications (neuropathy, renal disease, and retinopathy). The leading cause of mortality and morbidity in people with N1DDM is cardiovascular disease [108]. This is an acute or chronic increase in blood glucose concentration that results from decreased uptake of glucose into muscle and adipose tissues and increased hepatic glucose output. Several studies have demonstrated that even mild increases in chronic (fasting) or acute (postprandial) blood glucose concentration can contribute to macrovascular injury and atherosclerotic changes [109] .A close relationship has been established between poor glycemic control and the progression of retinopathy and polyneuropathy [110]. Conversely, intensive glycemic control prevents or significantly delays the development of nerve abnormalities and diseases related to microvascular changes in persons with NIDDM [110].

The mechanisms by which glucose produces its deleterious effects are not completely understood. However, the preponderance of evidence indicates that hyperglycemia increases oxidative stress, defined as the production of reactive oxygen species (free radicals; ROS) beyond the protective capability of the antioxidant defenses. The two primary mechanisms by which hyperglycemia may promote the generation of ROS are activation of the polyol pathway and increased glucose autooxidation. Enhanced ROS concentrations resulting from these mechanisms can cause general damage to proteins through cross-linking, fragmentation, and lipid oxidation. Reactive oxygen species may also mediate some of the changes associated with the development of atherosclerosis, for example, activation of coagulation, vasoconstriction, increased expression of adhesion molecules, and oxidative modification of low-density lipoprotein [111]. Increased uptake of glucose in the artery wall stimulates protein kinase C activity, which activates peroxidase enzymes and the cyclo-oxygenase pathway to produce an overabundance of ROS. In turn, these ROS may increase endothelial permeability, macrophage migration, and the secretion of endothelin, a cytokine believed to be involved in the development of atherosclerosis [108-110].

Another adverse effect of hyperglycemia is the nonenzymatic glycosylation of proteins. As a function of time and glucose concentration, protein amino groups react with glucose to eventually form advanced glycosylation end products (AGEs). The formation of AGEs often involves the participation of free radicals. Macrovascular and microvascular complications are the most common and significant consequences of glycosylation. The AGE-induced cross-linking of proteins in the vascular wall has been implicated in pathological changes associated with atherosclerosis, such as the accumulation of LDL particles [112]. The thickening, loss of elasticity, and increased permeability of blood vessel walls associated with microvascular complications may be due, in part, to glycosylation of vascular proteins[113].

There is now considerable evidence that hyperglycemia, hyperinsulinemia, and insulin resistance enhance free radical generation and thus contribute to oxidative stress in NIDDM [114]. Oxidative stress associated with hyperglycemia may lead to a reduced number of glucose transporters and impairment of insulin signaling [115]. Oxidative stress can even have adverse effects on β-cell insulin secretion. Therefore, oxidative stress resulting from hyperglycemia and insulin resistance can worsen

NIDDM by promoting further insulin resistance and decreased insulin secretion.

In obesity, a condition normally associated with NIDDM, there is increased oxidative stress that may be attributed to several mechanisms. A significant decline in insulin- mediated glucose uptake, which is often experienced by obese individuals, may result in hyperinsulinemia, which in turn may induce a rise in plasma free radical production. Hypertriglyceridemia and/or hypercholesterolemia observed in obese persons may facilitate the generation of ROS. It has been demonstrated that triglyceride-rich lipoproteins are more susceptible to oxidation, and that pro-oxidation kinetics and a decline in antioxidant effectiveness depend on LDL-cholesterol content [116]. In addition, the observation that obese rats on a calorie restricted diet have less oxidative stress than obese rats fed *ad labium* indicates that obesity is associated with an elevated degree of oxidative stress.

1.2.7.2. *Alteration of enzymatic antioxidant in diabetes mellitus*

Aerobic metabolism is always accompanied by the production of reactive oxygen species. Therefore, all aerobic organisms possess some sort of antioxidant defense, with enzymatic and non-enzymatic constituents [117].The quantity and quality of the reactive species is determined by metabolic pathways within the organism, influenced by exogenous factors such as radiation, food, stress, etc. The adverse effects of free radicals are recognized in several disorders [118], but care should be taken when assessing their causative role [119]. Damage caused by free radicals is possibly involved in β-cell destruction and in the pathogenesis of diabetes mellitus [120]. Alterations of metabolic processes in diabetes also influence enzymatic defenses, and these changes may be associated with late complications of diabetes. Antioxidant enzymes primarily account for intracellular defense, while several non-enzyme molecules, small molecule weight antioxidants, protect various components against oxidation in plasma (Fig. 1-14).

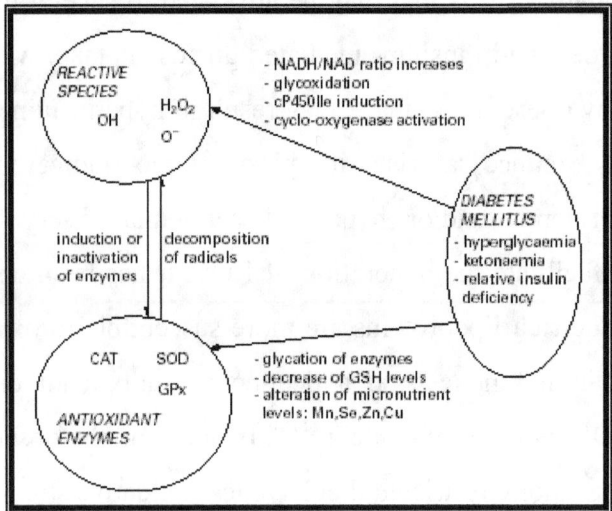

Figure 1-14. Suspected interaction between diabetes and antioxidant balance [117].

1.2.7.2.1. *The antioxidant enzymes*:

Antioxidant enzymes primarily provide intracellular antioxidant defense, which catalyze decomposition of reactive oxygen species. The three major antioxidant enzymes, superoxide dismutase (SOD), glutathione peroxidase (GPx), and catalase (CAT), differ from each other in structure, tissue distribution, and cofactor requirement. SOD catalyses the conversion of superoxide anion to hydrogen peroxide and oxygen. SOD activity was discovered by McCord and Fridovich in 1971; they later proved that the enzyme is required to sustain life in aerobic conditions [121]. Several classes of the enzyme have since been specified, each containing a transition metal in its catalytic center. In humans, mitochondrial MnSOD, and extra- and intracellular Cu/ZnSOD have been identified. Gpx is a selenium-dependent enzyme (selenoprotein). The extracellular form is a glycoprotein; the intracellular and mitochondrial forms also possess different antigenic structures. The substrate of the enzyme is reduced glutathione (GSH), and therefore it depends indirectly on the flavoprotein glutathione reductase (GRx) and cellular NADPH concentration. GPx uses a specific H donor, GSH, for the reduction of non-specific substrates (hydrogen peroxide, lipid and non- lipid hydroperoxides). The enzyme contains selenocystein in its active centre, which is incorporated into the polypeptide chain during translation. Selenium deficiency, both *in vitro* and *in vivo,* leads to enzyme deficiency. Thus, when assessing GPx function, it may be necessary to examine selenium status and free GSH concentration, at least when looking for the cause of altered activity [122].

Catalase is a haem-containing ubiquiter enzyme, in eukaryotes it is found in peroxisomes. The enzyme probably serves to degrade hydrogen peroxide produced by peroxisomal oxidase to water and oxygen. Several other enzymes are also involved in the prevention of oxidative damage or its repair, such as GRx, enzymes of NADPH production, and DNA repair enzymes. Different cell types and cellular compartments contain antioxidant enzymes in varying quantities. Regulation of antioxidant enzyme activity in eukaryote organisms may be influenced by such factors as age; hormonal state, organ specificity, and amount of cofactor present [122].

The metabolic alterations that accompany diabetes can affect pro-oxidant/antioxidant balance in several ways: induction, allosteric effects and activation/inactivation. Studies on experimental diabetes are carried out using certain spontaneously diabetic inbred animals or animals with viral or chemically induced diabetes [123]. Streptozotocin is a toxin which destroys beta-cells selectively; a single adequate dose produces lasting hyperglycaemia and insulin deficiency. It has been established that reactive free radicals have a role in this damaging effect [122]. Although the results of experimental animal studies cannot be extrapolated directly to human disease, this finding has raised questions on the etiologic role of free radicals in human diabetes.

1.2.7.2.1.1 *Superoxide Dismutase activity (SOD).*

In a long-term experiment Wohaieb (1987) observed a decrease of SOD activity in the liver and kidney and an increase in the pancreas of streptozotocin- treated diabetic rats and that increase in enzyme activity might be an adaptive response in the otherwise SOD-poor pancreas, while the reduction of SOD activity in liver and kidney might be due to the direct damaging effect of free radicals on the enzyme [124].

Dohi et al. (1988) found no difference in the SOD activity of the kidneys in streptozotocin treated diabetic rats after 4 months of diabetes [125] while, Matkovics et al. (1982) observed decreased SOD activities in all examined organs (liver, kidney, spleen, brain, heart, muscles, pancreas) except lungs of streptozotocin and alloxan treated diabetic rats[126] as well as Loven et al. (1986) observed a decrease in CuZnSOD activity in liver, kidney and erythrocytes after 10 days of streptozotocin-induced diabetes [127].

Sukalski et al. (1993) described the decrease of liver mitochondrial SOD activity [128]. A significant decrease of CuZnSOD activity in diabetic rabbit aorta endothelium was reported also by Tagami [129], although others have not found any difference in aortic SOD activity between diabetic and control rats [130]. Erythrocyte SOD activity is frequently measured in humans as an index of defense against superoxide in blood. In diabetes, activity of erythrocyte SOD has been shown to decreased, [126] increased [131] and unchanged [132-133].

Kawamura et al. (1992) showed that erythrocyte CuZn-SOD is glycated both in vitro and in vivo, leading to its inactivation, and the percentage of this glycated SOD is higher in IDDM children than in healthy individuals [134]. The percentage of extracellular glycated SOD has also been found to be higher in diabetes but its activity was comparable to that of the unmodified enzyme. Glycation was shown to affect the C-terminal end of the enzyme, reducing its heparin-binding affinity, thus, protection against extracellular radicals by cell-surface attached SOD may be impaired in diabetes, leaving the endothelium more susceptible to damage by superoxide anion [134].

1.2.7.2.1.2 *Glutathione peroxidase activity (GPx):*

Mukherjee et al. (1994) observed a significant reduction of GSH content after 15 years, and reduction of GRx activity after 3 weeks in liver, kidney, brain and blood of streptozotocin-treated diabetic rats [135]. Others have reported reductions in mitochondrial GPx and GRx activity in liver of diabetic rats [135].

Loven et al. studied intestinal mucosa and liver GSH content after 10 days of streptozotocin induced diabetes; there was a significant decrease of GSH in the liver while no change was noticed in the mucosa [127,136]. Orally administered GSH restored, and intramuscular insulin even raised liver GSH above normal levels. Abnormal GSH synthesis was thought to be responsible for the changes. Wohaieb SA et al (1987) found that in the liver, which normally contains high amounts of GSH and strong GPx activity, induction of diabetes caused a decrease in both, while in the kidney, which is relatively poor in GPx activity; diabetes led to an increase in activity, insulin reversed these alterations. GRx activity was shown to be increased in erythrocytes of spontaneously diabetic BB rats, while in alloxan-treated animals GPx activity was also increased [31,124]. The same group found similarly elevated erythrocyte GRx levels and resistance to peroxide-induced GSH reduction in type I and type II diabetic patients. They supposed that elevated glucose levels could increase NADPH production resulting in a more effective GSH reduction. Dohi T, (1988) noticed significant reduction in GPx activity in aorta homogenates of rats 4 and 8 months after the induction of diabetes. He found higher serum selenium concentrations in diabetic rats [125]. Tagami (1992) found reduced GSH content and Gpx activity and unchanged GRx activity in aortic endothelial cells of diabetic rabbits [129].

Langenstroer et al. (1992) found no alteration in GPx activity [130], but Blakytnye et al. (1992) observed that incubation of cow erythrocytes with glucose, glucose-6-phosphate and fructose results in a time-dependent reduction of GRx activity. The experiment suggested that glycation of the enzyme was responsible for the observed decrease. Decreased GRx activity in erythrocytes of diabetic children was reported by Stahlberg [137]), but Walter [138] found no difference between GPx and GRx activity of diabetics and non-diabetics. Mukherjee et al. (1994) examined erythrocytes of diabetics (fasting glucose > 140 mg/ml) and concluded that GSH reduction and glutathione elevation in erythrocytes caused by defective functioning of gammaglutamyl-cysteine synthase due to its glycation, decrease in GRx activity and defect in glutathione transport [135]. Yoshida et al. (1995) confirmed that in erythrocytes of poorly controlled diabetics (HbA_{1C} = 10.6 ± 1.3%) GSH synthesis and thiol transport is impaired, and cells become susceptible to oxidative damage [139].

Golden et al. (1988) found that erythrocyte GSH content was negatively correlated to HbA_{1C}, a good estimate of long-term hyperglycaemia, in diabetes. In diabetic patients with explicit hyperglycaemia (Hb A_{1C} = 11.5 ± 1.9). Uzel et al. (1987) found impaired GPx activity and lower erythrocyte GSH, in addition to elevated lipid peroxidation products, the alterations being more pronounced in patients with retinopathy [140].

Reduced GSH and protein-SH content in erythrocytes of diabetes was reported by Bono et al,[132] in addition to Kaji et al. reported no difference in erythrocyte GPx activity but an increase in plasma GPx activity of diabetic compared to non-diabetic women [133]. Elevation of serum selenium levels and GPx activity in diabetic children was reported by Cser [141]. Similarly, higher GPx activity has been reported in erythrocytes of diabetics by Matkovics et al [126].

1.2.7.2.1.3. Catalase activity (CAT)

Observations regarding catalase activity in the literature are rather controversial: a decrease, reversible by insulin, in aortic endothelial cell catalase activity in diabetic rabbits was reported by Tagami [129]. Dohi T, (1988) observed no alteration in catalase activity of rat aorta homogenate [150], while Langenstroer (1992) reported its elevation [130]. The activity of catalase in the liver and kidneys of diabetic animals is generally believed to decrease [124, 130], although there are also reports of its increase [125]. On the other hand, heart and pancreas tissues show increased catalase activity in the diabetic state [124].

Erythrocyte catalase activity seems not to be altered either in diabetic animals or in type 1 and 2 diabetic patients [124,130-133]. It is apparent from data mentioned above that contradictory changes in the activities of particular enzymes in particular organs have been observed in many cases. These discrepancies may be partly explained by the variability in the diabetes models used, including the strain and sex of the animals, their age at the induction of diabetes, the severity of the resulting insulin deficiency, and the duration of diabetes. For the clinical observations similar confounding factors exist, such as the type and duration of diabetes, mode of treatment, presence or absence of complications, which are not revealed by routine laboratory tests. Changes in enzyme activity (increased, impaired, unchanged) may depend on the above-mentioned factors to a large extent. [142]

Szaleczky et al. (1997) investigated that in type I diabetes, when blood glucose is strictly controlled by intensive insulin therapy, there is not accompanied by remarkable changes in the prooxidant-antioxidant balance, antioxidant enzyme activities (erythrocyte SOD and catalase, whole blood Gpx) do not differ from those of healthy controls [143].

In an investigation of the relationship between the duration of diabetes and various antioxidant activity in blood, Prechi J (1997) found that erythrocyte SOD was reduced in patients who had diabetes for more than 10 years compared to patients whose disease was not so long-standing, while whole blood GPx and erythrocyte catalase activities did not differ. In recent years it has been definitely shown that the worse the diabetic metabolic control, the higher the frequency of late complications [144].

Oxidative stress plays a role in the development of these complications. So researchers would expect adaptive changes to be observed in the antioxidant defense system. Presumably these changes would be of different magnitudes in different states of metabolic control and depend on the duration of the unfavorable metabolic state [144-145].

It is well-known that syndromes characterized by disturbances of carbohydrate metabolism are not a homogenous disease; the only common basis is that in all forms of diabetes there is an absolute or relative insulin deficiency. Previous studies have suggested that the clinical forms of late complications seem to be the same, although it has not been established whether the pathogenic factors involved in the development of the late complications are common and, if so, to what extent. If it is true that the oxidative stress has a role in the development of late complications, it is still not clear whether it has the same importance in the different forms of diabetes. Further, changes in carbohydrate metabolism may influence oxidative stress, the function of antioxidant defense and the damage caused. Keeping this in mind, investigations of the antioxidant system should include different types and degrees of disturbance of carbohydrate metabolism [143-146].

1.1.2.7.3. *Antioxidant based therapeutic approaches to NIDDM*

The body possesses defense mechanisms that, in the healthy individual, adequately control plasma reactive oxygen species (ROS) concentration under most conditions. However, in persons with NIDDM, increased plasma ROS generation and a marked reduction in antioxidant defenses result in oxidative stress, which in turn can lead to many of the deleterious effects of NIDDM. It is critical, therefore, that any therapies for NIDDM include the direct and/or indirect reduction of oxidative stress. As discussed previously, modifications of certain environmental factors, for example, exercise and especially weight loss can effectively prevent and even reverse the effects of NIDDM, in part by reducing oxidative stress [145-147].

Various hypoglycemic agents reduce oxidative stress, indirectly by lowering blood glucose levels and preventing hyperinsulinemia, and directly by acting as free radical scavengers. For example, gliclazide, a sulfonylurea normally used to augment insulin release, is an effective scavenger of superoxide and hydroxyl radicals. Recent studies have demonstrated that gliclazide can decrease LDL oxidation and monocyte adhesion to the endothelium, events that contribute to the development of atherosclerosis in NIDDM [148].

The insulin-sensitizing agent troglitazone also appears to possess some antioxidant activity. Antioxidant nutrients may complement the therapies described above to reduce oxidative stress. In general, exogenous antioxidants can compensate for the lower plasma antioxidant levels often observed in NIDDM and in pre-diabetic individuals, whether their diabetes is primarily genetic in origin or due to obesity and a sedentary lifestyle. It has long been suspected, but only recently demonstrated, that the consumption of fruits and vegetables rich in vitamin and other antioxidants can increase overall antioxidant status [174]. In studies of humans and rodents, dietary supplementation with antioxidants is associated with decreased risk of NIDDM and induces changes that could be beneficial in reducing insulin resistance and protecting vascular endothelium [150].

There is mounting evidence that a general increase in antioxidant status achieved by dietary supplementation can help diminish oxidative stress associated with NIDDM. However, certain antioxidants are of particular benefit with regard to the prevention and treatment of diabetic complications. Primary among these are vitamin E (α-tocopherol) and lipoic acid (thioctic acid). Vitamin E is a fat-soluble vitamin that effectively scavenges the peroxyl radical in cell membranes, thereby inhibiting lipid peroxidation. Prospective epidemiological studies demonstrate that high serum vitamin E levels are associated with decreased risk of NIDDM [151]. In the GK rat, a model for NIDDM, vitamin E supplementation significantly improves glycemic control, possibly by minimizing free radical damage to the pancreatic β-cells [152].

Improvements in glucose metabolism and insulin action in the obese Zucker rat, an animal that exhibits many of the features of NIDDM, may be mediated by a reduction in oxidative stress. Researchers found that glucose-stimulated hyperinsulinemia and lipid peroxidation in the obese Zucker rat could be significantly reduced with dietary vitamin E [152]. A similar finding has been observed in humans. Plasma concentrations of lipid hydroperoxides, an indicator of lipid peroxidation, were higher in healthy, insulin resistant volunteers has compared to insulin-sensitive ones, while plasma concentrations of vitamin E were significantly lower. Prospective studies of non-diabetic individuals provide evidence that vitamin E supplementation is associated with a protective effect against coronary heart disease [153].

In humans and in animal models of NIDDM, vitamin E reduces vascular oxidative stress and preserves endothelial function, thus inhibiting the development of atherosclerosis. Specifically, vitamin E supplementation by 400 µg per day can make LDL less susceptible to oxidation and consequently less atherogenic. Vitamin E supplementation has been demonstrated to prevent the induction of protein kinase C activity in the hyperglycemic aorta, thereby inhibiting the migration and proliferation of vascular smooth muscle cells. This effect of vitamin E can prevent or at least delay many of the vascular complications associated with NIDDM. Lipoic acid, an essential cofactor of alpha-oxoacid dehydrogenase complexes, is also a potent lipophilic free radical scavenger [154].

Several studies indicate that the decline in insulin mediated glucose uptake observed in NIDDM is due to oxidative stress, which in turn is associated with reduced glucose transporter (GLUT4) exposure and/or impairment of insulin signaling [155]. Lipoic acid was found to increase glucose transport in muscle cells in culture by stimulating translocation of GLUT4 from internal pools to the plasma membrane [150].

Antioxidant treatment has been demonstrated to prevent nerve dysfunction in experimental diabetes. Lipoic acid is of particular interest to researchers because it is a powerful free radical scavenger of peripheral nerves both in vitro and in vivo. It also promotes fiber regeneration and stimulates nerve growth factor. Several clinical studies reveal that lipoic acid is generally safe and effective in reducing symptoms of diabetic peripheral neuropathy. Short-term treatment for three weeks using 600 mg/day intravenously or 1800 mg/day orally appeared to reduce symptoms and improve neuropathic deficits [156]. Lipoic acid taken orally (600 mg/day) for 4-24 months reduced neuropathic deficits and improved motor and sensory nerve conduction in the lower limbs [156-158].

A number of other antioxidant nutrients have been reported to be beneficial for subjects with NIDDM. Flavonoids, a group of antioxidant polyphenolic compounds found ubiquitously in commonly consumed fruits and vegetables and in beverages, such as tea, have been demonstrated to protect against oxidative stress in type 1 and type 2 diabetes [184]. Specifically, the flavonoids inhibit lipid oxidation and delay the depletion of lipid-soluble antioxidants. Serum levels of carotenoids, another group of antioxidant compounds often present in edible plants, were inversely related to fasting serum insulin levels [160]. While not conclusive, this observation is suggestive of a role for carotenoids in the pathogenesis of insulin resistance and diabetes. Taurine and coenzyme Q10 are endogenous antioxidants that can also be obtained from the diet. In rats with diabetes induced by chemical destruction of β-cells, taurine supplementation (1% taurine in the drinking water) reduced renal oxidant injury by decreasing lipid peroxidation and inhibiting the accumulation of advanced glycation end products within the kidney [161]. The effects of oral treatment with coenzyme Q10 (60 mg twice daily) were examined in a randomized, double blind trial of 30 patients with coronary heart disease. After 8 weeks of treatment, the patients receiving coenzyme Q10 had reduced plasma levels of insulin (fasting and 2 hour), glucose, and lipid peroxides as compared to the control group [162]. These findings indicate that treatment with coenzyme Q10 in this group decreases oxidative stress and improves insulin sensitivity [162].

Aim of Thesis:

1. Evaluating the effect of crude and pure oleuropein in primarily animal studies on blood sugar, body weight and fluid intake using alloxan induced diabetic rabbit.

2. Determining the effect of pure oleuropein on lipid profile and uric acid in alloxan induced diabetic rabbits and in human non insulin dependent diabetes mellitus after long term administration.

3. Determining the effect of pure oleuropein after long administration on enzymatic antioxidant (SOD, G-6PD, CAT, GPx and GRx), and non-enzymatic antioxidant levels (vit. E, vit. C, and β-carotene) in addition to total antioxidant capacity in alloxan induced diabetic rabbits and human non insulin dependent diabetes mellitus.

4. Measuring the antimicrobial activity of oleuropein and its metabolites on different species of pathogenic bacteria isolated from patients attending hospitals.

5. Elucidating the effect of oleuropein intake on insulin receptors using lymphocyte cells as a model of binding study in non insulin dependent diabetes mellitus.

6. Studying the effect of oleuropein intake on beta cells in alloxan induced diabetic animals via histological study.

7. Studying the efficiency of using pure oleuropein as medicinal agent for the treatment of type 2 diabetes mellitus patients.

2.1 Chemicals, Instruments, and Samples

Chemicals Name & Supplied Company	
Acetic acid (BDH)	Kit for uric acid determination(BioMerieux)
Acetonitril (BDH)	Kit for Glucose determination(BioMerieux)
Acid Fuchin stain (Merck)	Kit for urea determination(BioMerieux)
Amino ethyl diphenyl borate (Merck)	Kit for Triglyceride determination(BioMerieux)
Apigenin (Extra-synthese)	Kit for HDL –c determination (BioMerieux)
Apigenin 7-glucoside (Extra-synthese)	Kit for total protein determination (Randox)
Ascorbic acid (BDH)	Kit for Bilirubin determination(Randox)
Bovine serum albumin (Randox)	Kit for GOT&GPT determination(Randox)
Butylated hydroxytolune (Randox)	Krebs- Ringer Solution (Sigma)
Caffeic acid (Extra-synthese)	LDL(Sigma)
Chloro dinitrobenzene (BDH)	L-Methonine(BDH)
Chloroform (BDH)	Luteolin (Extra-synthese)
Chlorogenic acid (Extra-synthese)	Luteolin 7-glucoside (Extra-synthese)
Collagenase (Sigma)	Lymphoprep (Sigma)
Copper sulphate(BDH)	Metaphosphoric acid(BDH)
Digitonin(BDH)	Methanol(BDH)
Diphenylamine(BDH)	Na-K titrate(BDH)
Dioxan(BDH)	Nitro blue tetrazolium (Sigma)
Dithiobis nitro benzoic acid(BDH)	Oleuropein (Extra-synthese)
EDTA sodium salt(BDH)	Oxidized GSH(BDH)
Eagles Medium (Sigma)	P-Coumaric acid (Extra-synthese)
Elenolic acid (Extra-synthese)	Phosphate buffer saline(BDH)
Ethanol (BDH)	Phosphotungestic acid (BDH)
Ethyl acetate (BDH)	Picric acid(BDH)
Ferulic acid (Extra-synthese)	Reduced GSH(BDH)
Folin-Ciocalteau Reagent (Sigma)	Riboflavin(BDH)
Formic acid(BDH)	Rutin (Aldrich)
Gallic acid (Aldrich)	Silica gel FOR TLC (Merck)
G-6-phosphate (Aldrich)	Silica gel For C. Chrom. (Merck)
Glutathione reductase (Sigma)	Sodium Azide(BDH)
Glycerol(BDH)	Sodiumdodecylsulphate(BDH)
Hematoxylin (Merck)	Sucrose(BDH)
Hexane(BDH)	Sinapic acid(Extra-synthese)
Hydrochloric acid(BDH)	Syringic acid(Extra-synthese)
Hydroxytyrosol (Extra-synthese)	Tocopherol acetate(BDH)
Insulin standard (Diasorin)	Triton x-100(BDH)
Insulin Labeled 125(Diasorin)	Trolox (Aldrich)
Isopropanol (BDH)	Tyrosol(Extra-synthese)
Kit For insulin (Diasorin)	Vanillic acid(Extra-synthese)
Kit For TEAC (Randox)	Verbascoside(Extra-synthese)
Kit for Cholesterol determination	Xylene (Aldrich)

Instruments

The instruments used in this work were LKB gamma counter type 1275 mini-gamma. Shimadzu UV–visible recorder spectrophotometer; Perkian–Elmer 60 MH_Z for NMR spectra; Rotary vacuum evaporator; Pye-Unicam SP3-100 for IR spectra. Panasonic 1330 microwave oven; Gallen kamp Incubator; Gallen kamp water bath; Gallen kamp Oven; Orion pH-meter, Metler Balance; Shimadzu LC-10AD(HPLC);Hitachi LC-25(HPLC); Digital Polarmeter; ELISA Model 200(Germany)

Plant Material

Experiments were carried out on olea *europaea* leaves of three varieties commonly cultivated in different area of Iraqi region. These varieties "were Labeeb and Al-Ashersy which originated locally, and Manzanillo is of Spanish origin as well as we selected Bid el Haman variety as control. Leaves were obtained from handpicked and collected at the end of March 2001 .Leaves dried on site in a Panasonic 1330 microwave oven, three times for 2 min at maximum power (2680W). Dried leaves were powdered and stored in a dry place in the dark. Several conditions were tested to extract oleuropein from *olea europaea* leaves. Oleuropein was extracted using water/alcohol at different volume ratios. Each extract was analyzed by TLC and HPLC to determine the amount of oleuropein, using pure oleuropein as a reference compound. Optimal conditions to extract oleuropein were repeated on leaves from the different three variety used in this study, in order to identify the best variety to use it as rich source of oleuropein in the present study.

2.2. Methods for producing extract of olive leaves

Patent of Nachman L (1998) was used for extraction of oleuropein from olive leaves [163]. In brief dried olive leaves powder (0.5 gm) was extracted twice with (5ml) either methanol, ethanol water, or various mixtures of methanol, ethanol and water. The effect of extraction time was examined over the range ½ to 24 hours at different temperatures (4, 25, 45, 60 and 75°C). The extracts were combined and diluted with water to produce solution with a minimum 20% aqueous content prior to washing with hexane (5 ml). The extract was then filtered through 0.45 µm filters and analyzed by TLC and HPLC.

2.2.1. Assay for total phenolic content in different variety of olive leaves extract.

The amount of total phenolic in olive leaf extracts was determined according to the Folin-Ciocalteu procedure [164], based on complex formation of molybdenum-tungsten blue with some modification to determine the total phenolic content in olive leaf extracts. The method is as follows: A stock solution of a solid composition according to the present extraction in 50% aqueous methanol is prepared. The stock solution is diluted with water to a concentration of about 200 to 250 µg/ml. Next, 20 µl of this solution is placed into each of three wells of a flat bottom ELISA plate. 100 µl of 0.1N Folin-Ciocalteu reagent (Sigma, diluted) is added to each of the same wells. After 0.5 to 5 minutes, 80 µl of aqueous sodium carbonate (75 g/L) is added to each well. The plate is incubated at room temperature for two hours. The optical density at 750 nm is measured. A calibration curve of six dilutions (20 µl each) of gallic acid with a concentration of 0-100 µg/ml is used (Figure 2-1). Using this assay, the total phenol content of the sample is expressed as an equivalent gallic acid (GAE).

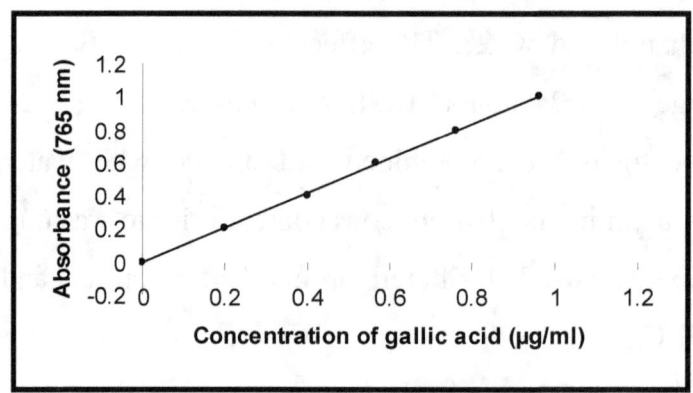

Figure 2-1. Calibration curve of gallic acid.

2.2.2. Rapid HPLC method for determination of oleuropein in olea europaea leaves [(165)]

HPLC analysis was performed on Shimadzu apparatus (two solvent delivery systems, automatic sample injector, tunable absorbance detector and photodiode array detector using symmetry C18, 5µm, 3.9 × 250 mm column). Data acquisition and quantitation were performed with Millennium 32, software. The mobile phase was 79% distilled water acidified (pH 3) with 0.1 M orthophosphoric acid (v/v, 1000:2.3) and 21 % acetonitril acidified with 0.1 M orthophosphoric acid (v/v ,1000:2.3). The flow rate was 1 ml/min and the injection volume was 20 µl. Routine quantitation of oleuropein was assessed at 280 nm. Run time was 35 min.

Samples for HPLC analysis carried out by extracting 5.0 gm of powdered leaves three times for 30 min with 30 ml of 50 % aqueous methanol, filtered solutions were mixed and diluted to 100 ml with the same solvent. Extracts were diluted (1:5) with mobile phase and added to an equal internal standard (coumarin 65 µg/ml) prepared with mobile phase.

TLC controls were performed on silica gel F_{254} (Merck) with chloroform /methanol/ acetic acid (70:30:10) plates were visualized under UV light at 254 nm and after ferric chloride solution (10%) had been sprayed for secoiridoids and amino ethyl diphenyl borate solution (10%) had been sprayed for flavonoids.

2.2.3. Optimization of extraction process (control)

Dried olive leaves (0.5 g) were blended with methanol/water (50/50, v/v; 5 ml) using an ultra high speed blender for 20 second. The solution was left to stand for 30 min and filtered using filter paper 0.45 µm. After hexane washing (5 ml), 1/3 of the extract by-mass was made up to a final mass of 3 gm with methanol / water (50/50, v/v); filtered through a 0.45 µm filter, and a portion injected into the chromatography. The remaining extract was stirred for 2 hour, and another third of the original extract was made up to 3 g with methanol/water (50/50, v/v) and filtered through a 0.45 µm filter, for subsequent HPLC analysis. The final third of the original extract was stirred, and after a total of 24 hour, was also made up to 3.0 g with methanol/water (50/50, v/v), filtered (0.45 µm) and analyzed by TLC and HPLC.

2.2.4. Acid and base hydrolysis

Dried olive leaves (0.5 g) were blended with methanol/water (50/50, v/v; 5 ml) using an ultra high speed blender for 20 sec. The solution was left to stand for 30 min and was filtered using 0.45 µm filter paper. After hexane washing (5 ml), hydrochloric acid (1 M, 2 ml) was added to the aqueous phase, and this solution was stirred for 2 hour. Half of the acidified extract was neutralized (pH 7) with NaOH (5 M), and the remaining extract was neutralized after 24 hour stirring. Both extracts were made up to a final mass of 3.0 g and were immediately filtered (0.45 μm) and analyzed by TLC and HPLC. The same procedure was used in the base hydrolysis experiments, however, NaOH (1 M, 2 ml) was added to the extract after hexane washing, and HCl (5 M) was used to neutralize the extracts after 2 and 24 hour, respectively.

2.2.5. Acid and base extraction

Dried olive leaves (0.5 g) were blended with methanol/water (50/50, v/v; 5 ml) using an ultra high speed blender for 20 sec. After standing for 30 min, hydrochloric acid (1 M; 2 ml) was added, and the solution was stirred for 2 hours. Half of the extract was filtered using 0.45 μm filter paper, and washed with hexane (5 ml). The aqueous extract was neutralized with NaOH (5 M), made up to a final mass of 3.0 g and filtered (0.45 μm) prior to analysis by HPLC. The remaining half of the extract was stirred for a total of 24 hour and was subjected to the same clean-up procedure as that of the 2 hour extract. The method above was also used for base hydrolysis experiments; however, NaOH (1 M, 2 ml) was added after standing the extract for 30 min, and HCl (5 M) was used to neutralize the extracts after 2 and 24 hour, respectively.

2.2.6. Separation of Phenolic compounds in methanolic leaves extract by RP-HPLC.

Separation was achieved on an ODS C18 column (5 μm, 150 mm x 4.6 mm) with gradient elution. Various gradients were compared but the three most suitable were based on those described by Servili et al. (1999) and Brenes et al. (1999) [166,167].

Gradient 1 (Servili. et al. 1999) used solvent A (water / acetic acid; 100/1, v/v) and solvent B (ethanol / acetonitril / acetic acid; 95/5/1, v/v/v) with a 2 min isocratic elution (5% solvent B) followed by a stepwise linear increase to 100% solvent B at 45 min.

Gradient 2 (Brenes et al. 1999) used methanol as solvent A with water / acetic acid (0.02%) as solvent B.

Gradient 3 employed the same solvents as for gradient 1 but with a much shallower gradient comprising a linear increase from 10% to 30% solvent B at 10 min followed by a 5 min isocratic elution and then linear increases to 40% solvent B (at 25 min), 50% at 40 min and 100% at 50 min with a final 5 min isocratic run and return to initial conditions over 25 min.

Table2-1.Gradient elution programs used for RP-HPLC

Time(min)	Solvent A(ml)	Solvent(B(ml)
Gradient 1		
0.0	20	80
30	80	20
35	80	20
50	100	0.0
55	100	0.0
Gradient 2		
0.0	85	15
12	85	15
35	66	34
40	85	15
Gradient 3		
0.0	80	20
5.0	80	20
35	20	80
37	0.0	100
40	0.0	100
42	80	20

2.2.7. *Large scale preparation of olive leaves extract by optimized conditions:*

For large scale preparation , leaves of the tree *Olea europaea* were tested for oleuropein content using thin layer chromatography and high pressure liquid chromatography, Approximately 1 kilogram of leaves is covered with 3.8 liters of (3:1v/v) ethanol solution in water, and the leaves remain covered at 60°C for 4 hours. At the end of the 4 hour period, the alcohol is drained and another 3.8 liter portion of (3:1v/v) ethanol is used to cover the leaves. This procedure is repeated twice more, and after the fourth cover, all extracts were combined and distilled under vacuum to produce a concentrated alcoholic solution containing about 25% to 30% solids. The solution dried to obtain a dry powder extract containing about 30% oleuropein. It may be desirable to conduct such steps at a temperature no greater than about 88 C° to avoid degradation of the glucoside. The oleuropein can then be purified, for example, by chromatographic separation procedures.

2.3. Isolation and purification of oleuropein from olive leaves extract:

2.3.1. *Isolation of oleuropein from olive leaves extract by column chromatography:*

A method of Garibaldi (1986) was used for isolation of oleuropein from olive leaves [168]. In brief, (500 gm) of powdered *olea europeae* leaves (Labeeb variety) were extracted with 75 % aqueous ethanol. After evaporation of ethanol, the aqueous phase was extracted with chloroform. Phenolic compounds were extracted with ethyl acetate. The ethyl acetate phase was totally evaporated to obtain 23.5 gm dried extract, (6.0) gm was separated by column chromatography using 200 gm silica gel 60 (Merck, 70-230 mesh) and eluting with 1 liter of chloroform-methanol (9:1), then with 400 ml of chloroform-methanol (4:1). Combined fractions gave 5.0 gm oleuropein. The first fractions of this chromatography 750 mg were chromatographed using 50 gm silica gel and eluting with 900 ml chloroform-methanol (99:1) then with 400 ml of chloroform-methanol (9:1). Combined fraction gave 150 mg hydroxytyrosol as less polar compound 50 mg oleoside and 120 mg verbascoside. Identification was established using, TLC, UV, IR and NMR compared to those reported in the literature.

2.3.2. Isolation of oleuropein from olive leaves extract by RP-HPLC:

A method of Cyril (2001) was used for isolation oleuropein from olive leaves [169]. In brief, 500 gm of powdered *olea europeae* leaves (Labeeb variety) were extracted with 50% aqueous methanol. After evaporation of methanol, the aqueous phase was extracted with chloroform. Phenolic compounds were extracted with ethyl acetate, the ethyl acetate phase was totally evaporated to obtain 23 gm dried extract, 5.0 g of the extract was subjected to low pressure liquid chromatography on chromatospac Prep 10 with a 40 × 500 mm column filled with Lichropep RP-18 (25-40µm) , 200 g Merck).The gradient solvent system was methanol /water (v/v,) 35:65 (500ml); 40:60 (500ml); 45:55 (500 ml); 70:30 (500 ml); 100:0 (1000 ml). Collected fractions (100 ml) each were examined by TLC. Five compounds were isolated: rutin, and luteolin 7–glucoside (35%) methanol fractions, verbascoside in the 40% methanol fractions, oleuropein in the 45 % methanol fractions and oleuroside in the 70% methanol fractions

Identification was established using TLC, UV, IR and NMR compared to those reported in the literature.

2.3.3. Isolation and purification of oleuropein by Preparative TLC:

Preparative thin-layer chromatography (PTLC) was conducted on glass plates (20 x 20 cm) coated with silica gel 50 F254. The ethyl extract (100 µL) was applied to the origins of 10 plates, and these were developed in the mobile phase methanol-water-acetic acid (50:50:1), by volume. Bands on the thin-layer chromatography plates were detected under ultraviolet (UV) light (254 nm), and where relevant were scraped from the plates, pooled, and extracted three times with ethyl acetate. Solvent was removed under vacuum pressure. The residue is spray dried to obtain a dry powder extract oleuropein. It may be desirable to conduct such steps at a temperature no greater than about 88 C° to avoid degradation of the glucoside.

2.4 Preparation of oleuropein aglycone:

Limiroli (1995) method was performed for oleuropein enzymatic hydrolysis by β-glucosidase to obtain glucose and oleuropein aglycone [170]. 100 mg of β-glucosidase enzyme (from almonds) was added to a solution of 50 ml of phosphate buffer (pH 7.0) containing five gram oleuropein. The reaction mixtures were incubated at 60°C and the reaction time course was followed for three hour. The drawn samples were screened by TLC using as eluent a mixture of chloroform/methanol (8:2, v/v). Extraction of the aglycone was carried out with 100 ml of chloroform/methanol (2/l; v/v) and the organic phase was evaporated to dryness under nitrogen, purity of the extract was checked by TLC and HPLC using an RP-C18 column (250 ×4.6 mm) under the conditions described by Limiroli UV, IR and NMR spectral data were compared with that reported by the literature [170].

2.5. Preparation of elenolic acid:

Acid hydrolysis of oleuropein aglycone was carried out as described by Garibaldi [168]. Two grams of oleuropein aglycone was treated with 1 M sulphuric acid (15 ml), and dioxan (15 ml) was added to dissolve the sample and the mixture left 40 C for 6 hours. After this period, the dioxan was evaporated under vacuum, sodium bicarbonate was added and the solution was extracted with ethyl acetate. The aqueous phase was treated with 1 M HCL then extracted with chloroform (5×15ml), after drying and solvent evaporation, 500 mg of crude elenolic acid was obtained. The crude was chromatographed on silica gel (10 g) eluting with chloroform-isopropanol (49:1) + 1% HCOOH (TLC were run in the same eluent (× 3) and the acid-enriched fractions (200 mg) purified on silica gel (10 g) eluting with chloroform-isopropanol (99:1) + 1 % HCOOH to give 150 mg elenolic acid with UV maximum at 237 nm.

2.6. Biological activity of OLE

2.6.1. LDL oxidation test

LDL oxidation (ox-LDL) test was performed as previously described by Balla [171'], with slight modifications. In brief, 1.0 ml LDL solution (200 mg protein) was incubated with 1.0 ml copper sulfate (final concentration, 5 µM) as oxidizing agent during three time periods (1, 3, and 6 hours at 37°C) in shaking water bath and oxidation was terminated by refrigeration at 4C and addition of 0.1 mmol/l Na$_2$EDTA to chelate the copper ions. LDL oxidation was determined immediately by measuring the formed amounts of thiobarbituric acid-reactive substances (TBARS), mainly malonaldehyde (MDA), spectrophotometrically at 532 nm, after reaction with thiobarbituric acid solution [172]. An ox-LDL-blank test was also performed in the absence of copper ions. Each test was carried out three times. Determination of serum MDA was carried out by the addition of 1 ml of 17%TCA solution and 1ml of (0.6%) TBA solution to the all serum tube at different concentration of phenolic compounds then, all tubes were boiled at 100 C for 15 minutes. After cooling, 1 ml of 70% TCA solution was added, centrifuge for 15 minutes and take the supernatant and read at 532 nm.

$$\text{Conc. of MDA} = \frac{\text{Absorbance of the test at 532 nm}}{1.56 \times 10^5} \times \text{d.f}$$

2.6.2. Inhibition of LDL oxidation test

The inhibitory effect of the tested compounds (oleuropein, luteolin-7-glucoside, hydroxytyrosol, rutin) was estimated using the ox-LDL test with simultaneous addition of each material, diluted in 0.01 ml ethanol and 0.99 ml copper sulfate (instead of 1.0 ml copper sulfate) as oxidizing agent. Each substance was examined three times. Because of this number of replications, only simple descriptive statistics were used. Finally, the protection activity, expressed as percent mean protection (% MP), was assessed, after taking into consideration the ox-LDL. TBARS values with respect to LDL autooxidation as indicated by the ox-LDL -blank test.

2.6.3. Inhibition of erythrocytes hemolysis induced by AAPH. [173]

Blood samples were obtained from the rabbit ear vein. The erythrocytes were separated from plasma by centrifugation at 2500 rpm for 10 min. The crude erythrocytes were then washed three times with five volumes of phosphate buffered saline (PBS, pH 7.4). The packed erythrocytes were then suspended in four volumes of PBS solution. Oxidative hemolysis in erythrocytes induced by a peroxyl radical initiator, 2,2-azo-bis-(2-amidinopropane) dihydrochloride (AAPH), was chosen as a model for the peroxidative damage in biomembrane. Addition of AAPH to a suspension of erythrocytes caused oxidation of lipids and proteins in cell membrane and thereby induced hemolysis. The AAPH-induced hemolysis in RBC is a function of incubation time and is proportional to the concentration of free radicals. The inhibitory effect against erythrocytes hemolysis is also proportional to the concentration of antioxidants in the incubation mixture. Two milliliters of RBC suspension was mixed with 2 ml of PBS solution containing varying amounts of polyphenolic compounds (oleuropein; hydroxytyrosol; luteolin-7-glucoside elenolic acid, rutin, and Trolox as control). One milliliter of 400mM AAPH in PBS solution was then added to the mixture. The incubation mixture was shaken gently in a water bath at 37 °C for 3 h. After incubation, 8 ml of PBS solution was added into the reaction mixture followed by centrifugation at 3000 rpm for 10 min. The absorbance (A) of the supernatant at 540 nm was recorded in a Shimadzu 1201 spectrophotometer. Percentage inhibition was calculated by the following equation:

$$\% \ Inhibition = (A_c - A_t)/A_c$$

In which A_t is the absorbance of the sample containing glucoside and A_c is the absorbance of the control.

2.6.4. Assay of radical scavenging activity of oleuropein:

The radical scavenging activity of phenolic compounds was evaluated according to Re et al. (1999) [174]. This method is based on the ability of antioxidant to scavenge the stable ABTS radical cation, a blue/green chromophore with characteristic absorbance at 734 nm, in comparison to that of Trolox (a water-soluble tocopherol analogue). ABTS in water (7 mM) was mixed with potassium persulphate (2.45 mM) and allowed to react by standing in the dark at room temperature for 15 h. before use. The ABTS radical cation solution was then diluted with ethanol to an absorbance of 0.70 (± 0.02) at 734 nm and equilibrated at 30 °C. After addition of aliquots of Trolox or sample solutions to 1.0 ml of this diluted solution, the absorbance reading was taken at 30 °C exactly 1 min after initial mixing.

The extent of decolorization was expressed as percentage inhibition of the ABTS radical cation absorbance and plotted as a function of concentration of antioxidants. The activity of each compound was determined at four concentrations, within the range of the dose response curve of Trolox and the Trolox equivalent antioxidant capacity (TEAC), defined as the concentration (mmol/L) of Trolox having the equivalent scavenging activity to a 1.0 mM solution of the substrate under investigation, and was calculated. All determinations were carried out twice at each separate concentration of the samples.

2.6.5. The effect of oleuropein on glucose uptake in isolated fat cells [175]

Materials

1-Sodium chloride (0.154 mol/1)

2-Potassium chloride (0.154 mol/1)

3-Calcium chloride (0.110 mol/1)

4-potassium phosphate (0.154 mol/1)

5-Magnesium sulphate (0.154 mol/1)

6-Sodium bicarbonate (0.154 mol/1)

7-Krebs-Ringer bicarbonate with reduced calcium concentrations (KRB). Solutions 1-6 were in the following proportions then gas with 95% O_2 /5%CO_2 for 20 min.

Solution No	Volume (ml)
1	100
2	4.0
3	1.5
4	1.0
5	1.0
6	21

8- KRB-albumin solution: a 30 % w/v solution of albumin in KRB was prepared and dialyzed overnight against KRB in the cold .then after 24 hours diluted to 4% w/v albumin with KRB and gassed to pH 7.4 with 95% O_2 / 5% CO_2 and stored at 37 C in a sealed container under an atmosphere of 95% CO_2.

9- Incubation medium (KRB-albumin containing 3 mmol/1 glucose)

10- Gas cylinder of 95% O_2/5%CO_2

11- Male rabbit (750-1000g)

12-Plastic tubes (10-15 ml)

13- Collagenase (3 mg).

14- Shaking water bath at 37 C.

Methods

<u>Preparing of isolated fat cells</u>: One male rabbit was killed and the two epididymal fat pads were removed and placed in 10 ml of KRB -albumin containing 3 mg of collagenase in a plastic tube, then gassed briefly with 95%O_2/5%CO_2, sealed the tube, and incubated by shaking for 1 hour in a 37C water bath. Any tissue fragments was removed with forceps and the cell suspension was centrifuged in a plastic centrifuge tube at 400 g for 1 min, then penterated the layer of fat cells on the surface with a pasture pipette and removed the infranantant and sedimented cells by aspiration.The fat cells were resuspended in a 10 ml of KRB - albumin and washed by gentle stirring with plastic rods, centrifuged at 400 g for 1 min and again removed and discard the infranatant. The washing procedure was repeated twice more and finally the cells were resuspended in a suitable volume of the incubation medium (KRB-albumin-glucose).

Glucose uptake:

First, the dose response curve for the stimulation of glucose uptake by insulin was determined by incubating 1 ml of the fat cell suspension in triplicate with the following final concentrations of insulin, 0.0; 1.0; 10.0; 100.0; 1000 micro unit /ml (1 mg= 25 units). The insulin was added in a small volume (5 μl) to the plastic incubation tubes followed by 1 ml aliquots of the stirred cell suspension using a wide bore 1ml plastic syringe, then gassed with 95%O_2/5%CO_2 for 2 min and incubated in sealed plastic tubes for 2 hours at 37 °C with gentle shaking. After incubation, the cells were centrifuged and the glucose remaining in the incubation medium was determined using the glucose assay by Tinder method [177]. The results were expressed as a mean number of micromoles of glucose taken up per milliliter of suspension per hour ± standard error of the three incubations. A graph of glucose uptake (μmol/ml/h) against insulin concentration was plotted to give the dose response curve. This experiment was repeated in the presence of different concentration of oleuropein. (0, 20, 40, 60, 80 and 100 μmol/L).

2.7. Animal Studies

2.7.1. Animal design:

All animals used in this work were Newzeland male rabbits purchased from Al-Razzi center for diagnostic kits research in Baghdad. Male rabbit (850-1000 g weight) were used at 3 month age .Groups of rabbits were housed at room temperature with a lighting schedule of 12 hrs light and 12 h dark. Animals had free access to a standard pellet diet and tap water.

2.7.2. Induction of diabetes:

Animals were rendered diabetic by treatment with alloxan intravenously in a daily dose of 150 mg/kg for 1 week. By the end of that period, the animals showed a significant rise in blood sugar, the blood sugar was measured non-invasively at weekly intervals. At least 3 readings of blood sugar were taken for each animal and the mean value were calculated

2.7.3. Prophylactic antihyperglycemic effect of crude oleuropein:

In order to investigate the potential usefulness of the extract in preventing the development of diabetes induced by alloxan, three groups of rabbits, 8 animals each, were randomly divided into the following groups:

1- *Control group*: animals received no extract medication, but were given an oral dose of soy oil (0.2 ml) daily for 16 weeks.

2- *Alloxan treated rabbits group*: animals were treated with alloxan intravenously in a daily dose of 150 mg/ Kg for one week. No medical treatment for 4 weeks but were given an oral dose of soy oil (0.2 ml) daily for 4 weeks.

3- *Alloxan+ oleuropein treated groups*: Animals were treated with alloxan for week as above, but with the concomitant administration of crude oleuropein (Ethyl acetate extract of olive leaves) in doses of 25, 50 and 100 mg/kg for the same length of time. The extract was given orally as an powdered form prepared shortly before use with (0.2 ml) soy oil as carrier. The body weight and fluid intake of all animals were recorded on a weekly basis as described above.

Alloxan solution: 150 mg/ kg dissolved in normal saline and injected intravenously by 1.0 ml disposable syringe, alternatively a 20 % solution of glucose injected intraperitoneal after 4-6 hr. repeat this process 5 days. After 7 days of treatment by alloxan the glucose levels was determined [176]

2.7.4 Effect of oleuropein administration in diabetic rabbits:

In order to study whether or not the oleuropein is capable of reducing the blood sugar of rabbits with established diabetes, rabbits were rendered diabetes by daily intravenously administration of alloxan for 1 week. Animals were allocated to the following groups.

1- *Control group:* eight animals were used in this group. They received no mediation but were given an oral dose of soy oil (0.2ml) daily for the duration of the experimental period (16 weeks).

2- *Diabetic group*: Sixteen animals were included in this group. The rabbits rendered diabetes by treatment with alloxan intravenously in a daily dose of 150 mg/ kg for one week; they received no medication but were given an oral dose of soy oil (0.2 ml) daily for the duration of the experimental period (4 weeks). Then the animals were randomly divided into two groups each group contain eight rabbits .First group was given crude oleuropein in a daily oral dose of 20 mg/ kg for the next 16 weeks while second group was given pure oleuropein in a daily oral dose of 20 mg/kg for the next 16 weeks. All biochemical assays were carried out on all two groups before and after treatment compared with healthy group.

2.7.5. Toxicity of oleuropein:

Twenty-five healthy rabbits divided into five groups, each group were administrated orally a gradient increasing dose of crude oleuropein daily for 16 weeks period started from 1, 2, 3, 4, and 5 gm against control group . Fasting blood samples were carried out weekly for determination of total serum bilirubin, serum GOT, and serum GPT, serum ALP, serum total protein, serum albumin, blood urea, and serum creatinine until the end period of experiment (16 weeks) and the results were evaluated.

2.8. Human study

2.8.1. NIDDM group:

Thirty male patients with type 2 diabetes (NIDDM), volunteered for this study. (Mean age 55 ± 10 years).We hypothesized that the degree of oxidative stress and unbalanced of antioxidant levels would have a parallel trend. Because such a trend could be better shown in patients with elevated oxidative stress, we determined that patients with type 2 diabetes would be the best. Glucose metabolic control was assessed by measuring glycated hemoglobin (Hb A_{1C}). All tests were performed in the morning after the subjects had fasted overnight. Each treatment lasted 6 months. We selected 6 months because in our previous studies (animal study) we found that this length of time is necessary to observe any effect of olive leaf extract. At the end of the treatment period the patients were evaluated.

2.8.2. Healthy subjects:

Twenty five healthy male volunteers (mean age 45 ± 7 years) were studied. Health was defined as an absence of major medical or surgical illness during the previous 5 years with no hospital admission, current medication, or a subjective perception of good health.

2.8.3. Blood Sampling:

Blood samples both in human or animal studies were drawn in the fasting state and processed within 1 hour of collection. Samples were centrifuged for 5 min at 1500 g, and then plasma and Buffy-coat were removed by aspiration. Erythrocytes were washed three times with phosphate buffered saline (PBS), pH (7.4); 0.02M phosphate; 0.123 M NaCl. The packed erythrocyte volume (PCV) after the final wash was used for the assay of GSH, GPx, GRx, HbA_{1C}, G-6-PD, and MDA. Serum or plasma was stored at (-20C) and used later for other biochemical parameters required.

2.9. Biochemical assays

2.9.1. *Determination of blood sugar:*

A standard enzymatic method by Tinder [177] was used for determination of glucose spectrophotometrically at 500 nm.

2.9.2. Determination of Hemoglobin

Hemoglobin was determined in whole blood and hemolysate by the method of cyanomethemoglobin using Drabkin reagent [178] of commercially available kit (Randox Laboratories UK).

2.9.3. *Determination of glycated hemoglobin (HbA1C):*

A standard colorimetric method reported by Standderfor [179] was used to determine the glycated hemoglobin .The principle of this method depends on transform a glucose group in Hb to the 5-hydroxy methyl furfural at high temperature and pressure at acidic conditions, so this compound reacts with thiobarbituric acid (TBA) to form a colored complex compound measured spectrophotometrically at 443 nm.

Assay:

2.8 ml of distill water was added to 0.2 ml of red blood cells, mixed well then the conc. of hemoglobin was measured in the hemolysate by Drabkin's method [178]. Seven tubes were prepared: one for Test and the second to the Blank, and the other five tubes for the standard fructose solution. 1 ml of 0.5 M oxalic acid solution was added to all tubes. Tubes were tightly closed and autoclaved for 60 min. After cooling the tubes 1 ml of 40% TCA solution was added to each tube, mixed well, then T and B tubes were centrifuged and 1.5 ml of supernatant add to 0.5 ml of TBA (except Blank tube). All tubes were heated at 40°C for 10 minutes. A calibration curve was plotted between the conc. of fructose standards and the absorbance at 443 nm (Figure 2-2).

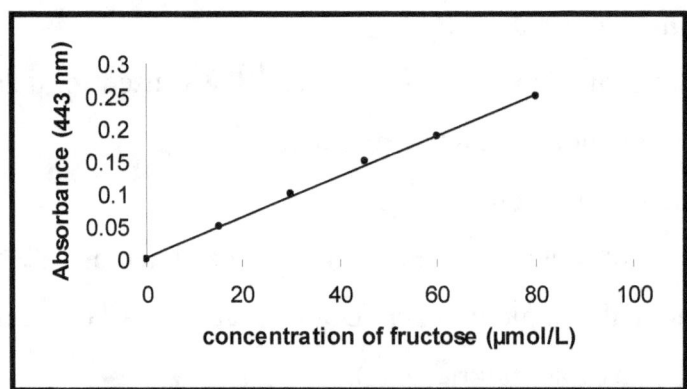

Figure 2-2. Calibration curve of fructose determination.

Calculation:

Hb (µmol/L) =   Conc. of Hb (g/dl) x d.f. x 1000/64

HbA_{1c} % = (HbA_{1c}/ Hb) x 100

2.9.4. *Determination of serum total cholesterol:*

Total concentration of cholesterol was measured by enzymatic method of Richmond [180], with commercially available kit (bioMerieux France). Total cholesterol is determined spectrophotometrically at 500 nm.

2.9.5. *Determination of serum high density lipoprotein (HDL-c):*

HDL-c was measured by enzymatic method of Burstein [181] with commercially available kit (bioMerieux-France). The principle of this method is to precipitate the chylomicrons and lipoproteins of very low density lipoprotein (VLDL) and low density lipoprotein by the addition of phosphotungestic acid in the presence of magnesium ion. The supernatant obtained after centrifugation contained high density lipoprotein (HDL) from which the cholesterol and phospholipids can be determined. High density lipoprotein is determined spectrophotometrically at 500 nm.

2.9.6. *Determination of serum triglycerides:*

Total serum triglycerides concentration was measured by enzymatic method of Fossati [182] with commercially available kit (BioMerieux France). Total serum concentration of triglycerides was determined at 500 nm.

2.9.7. *Determination of serum very low density lipoprotein (VLDL-c):*

Very low density lipoprotein was determined according to the conventional Friedewald equation [183].

$$VLDL\text{-}c \ (mg/dl) = 0.2 \ x \ TG \ (mg/dl)$$

2.9.8. *Determination of serum low density lipoprotein (LDL-c):*

Serum low density lipoprotein is determined according to Friedewald equation [183].

$$LDL\text{-}c = T\text{-}Chol. - (HDL\text{-}c + VLDL\text{-}c)$$

2.9.9. Determination of serum uric acid determination:

Serum uric acid was measured by enzymatic method of Artiss JD [184] with commercially available kit (bioMerieux.France). Serum uric acid was determined at 520 nm.

2.9.9. Determination of blood urea:

Blood urea was measured by enzymatic method of Chaney [185] with commercially available kit (bioMerieux.France).Blood urea was determined at 500 nm.

2.9.11. Determination of serum creatinine:

Serum creatinine was measured, after deproteinization; according to the jaffe reaction [186] using commercially available kit (biomerieux .France) .Serum creatinine was measured at 520 nm.

2.9.12. Determination of total serum protein:

Total serum protein was measured on the principle of the Biuret reaction [187] using available commercially kit (biomerieux, France). Serum protein was measured at 540 nm.

2.9.13. Determination of serum albumin:

Serum albumin was measured on the principle of its quantitative binding to the indicator bromocresol green at 578 nm using commercially available kit from Randox (England) [188].

2.9.14. Determination of serum total bilirubin:

Total serum bilirubin was measured on the principle of diazo-reaction [189] with sulfanilic acid at 540 nm, using commercially available kit (Randox).

2.9.15. Determination of serum GOT activity:

Serum GOT activity was measured colorimetric ally according to the Reitman and Frankle method [190] using a commercially available kit (Randox).

2.9.16. Determination of serum GPT activity:

Serum GPT activity was measured colorimetrically according to the Reitman and Frankle method [190] using a commercially available kit (Randox).

2.9.17. Determination of serum alkaline phosphatase activity (ALP):

Serum ALP activity was measured colorimetric ally according to Belfield [191], using a commercially available kit (bioMerieux.France)

2.9.18. Erythrocyte and plasma malondialdehyde (MDA) assay:

Malondialdehyde (MDA) was assayed according to the method of Ohkawa [192] with minor modification. The reaction to form thiobarbituric acid reactive substances (TBARs) depends on the condensation of two molecules of TBA with one molecule of MDA to generate a reddish chromogen that absorb light at 532nm wave length.

Assay

0.1 ml of plasma or erythrocyte suspension was transferred to screwed-cap Pyrex tube. 0.1 ml of 8.1 % SDS, 0.75 ml of 20% acetic acid solution and

0.75 ml of 0.8%aqueous solution of TBA were then added to the sample. All samples included butylated hydroxytoluene (BHT) (10µl:99mg/10ml absolute alcohol) to avoid auto-oxidation when exposed to high temperature. The mixture was made up to 2.0 ml with D.W., homogenized, and heated in a water bath at 95°C for 60 min. After cooling, 2.5 ml of n-butanol /pyridine (15:1) and 0.5 ml D.W. were added, vortex vigorously and centrifuged at 3000 rpm for 15 min. The TBARs was measured by following the increase in absorbance at 532 nm in the n- butanol/pyridine phase. Blank includes all the assay mixture except TBA.

Calculations:

Hemoglobin was determined for the original cell-suspension and calculation was performed using the formula.

$$\text{\textit{Erythrocyte MDA conc. (µmol/g Hb)}} = \frac{A \times D.F.}{\xi \times d \times Hb\ (g/L)}$$

A: Absorbance,

d.f.: Dilution factor = 25,

ξ: Extinction coefficient = 1.56×10^5 M^{-1}.cm^{-1}

Hb: hemoglobin concentration (g/L).

d: light path = 1 cm

2.9.19. Erythrocyte glucose 6-phosphodehydrogenase (G6PD) assay:

Measurement of G6PD activity was performed according to the method of Tietz [193] which is a modified version of Bishop (1966). G6PD catalyzes the oxidation of G-6-P to form 6-PG with the conversion of NADP to NADPH. The increase in absorbance due to NADPH formation is followed at 340nm wavelength and it is a function of enzyme activity.

A) *Reagents*:

1) Digitonin 0.01 mg/dl D.W.

2) Reaction mixture solution: 1.82 mg of Tris-(hydroxymethyl) amino methane was dissolved in 80ml D.W. at 37°C then the pH was adjusted to 8.0 with 6N HC1. 0.304gm of $MgCl_2.6H_2O$; 0.023gm of NADP (Na)-salt and 0.030gm of G-6-P (Na)-salt were dissolved in Tris buffer and the volume was completed to 100 ml with D.W. 2.0 ml aliquot was pipette into test tubes, the tube contents and the aliquots were kept in the freezer (-20°C). The aliquots were stable for 6-8 weeks (Tietz, 1984) [215].

B) *Assay*:

1) 1.0 ml of digitonin solution was Pipette to a test tube.

2) 0.01 ml of erythrocyte suspension was added to the digitonin solution and mix to hemolyze.

3) The hemolysate and the tube containing assay mixture were Incubate in water bath at 37°C for 10 min)

4) The hemolysate was transfer to the assay mixture and inverted several times to mix.

5) The absorbance was measured at 340nm.

6) The assay system was reincubated for l0 min at 37°C and the absorbance was measured again to obtain Δ A.

7) Hemoglobin concentration for the original erythrocyte suspension was measured.

8) Blank tube was contained 2.0ml reaction mixture plus 1.0 ml digitonin solution plus 0.01ml D.W. or Saline.

C) Calculations:

$$G\text{-}6PD \text{ activity in RBC } (U/g\ Hb) = \frac{\frac{\Delta A}{t} \times V_t \times 1000}{\xi \times Vs \times d \times Hb(g/L)}$$

Δ A: Difference in absorbance

V_t : Total volume of assay=3.01

V s: sample volume = 0.01 ml

ξ: Extinction coefficient = 6.22 mM $^{-1}$. Cm^{-1}

d: Length of light path = 1.0 cm

Hb: Hemoglobin concentration in hemolysate.

t: time interval (10min).

2.9.20. Erythrocyte glutathione (GSH) assay:

Glutathione was assayed with a method of Beutler [194]. Virtually all of the no protein sulfohydryl groups of RBCs are in the form of reduce glutathione. 5.5-Dithiobis-(2-nitrobenzoic acid), DTNB, is a disulfide chromogen that is readily reduced by sulfohydryl compounds to intensively yellow compound. The absorbance of the reduced chromogen is measured at 412nm and is directly proportional to the GSH concentration.

A) Reagents:

1) Precipitating solution: 30gm NaCl, 0.02gm EDTA, and 1.67gm glacial Metaphosphoric acid. All these substance were dissolved in 100ml D.W. The mixture was stable for 3 weeks at 4°C.

2) Na_2HPO_4 solution (0.3M). 42.59gm of Na_2HPO_4 was dissolved in 1L D.W.

3) 40mg of DTNB was dissolved in 100ml of 1% trisodium citrate solution. The mixture was stable for 13 weeks at 4°C.

B) Assay:

1) 0.2ml of erythrocyte suspension was placed into 1.8ml D.W. and mixed to hemolyze.then 3.0 ml of MPA solution was promptly added, mixed and Leaved to stand for 5min at room temperature then filtered through coarse-grade filter paper.

4) Cuvetts as follow were prepared:

Reagent	Test (ml)	Blank (ml)
1 .Filtrate	0.5	-----
2.MPA	----	0.3
3.H$_2$0	----	0.2
4.Na$_2$HP0$_4$	2.0	2.0
5.DTNB	0.25	0.25

5) Absorbance was measured with in 3min of preparing cuvetts.

6) Hb concentration was determined for the original cell suspension.

C) Calculation:

$$Erythrocyte\ GSH\ (\mu mol/g\ Hb) = \frac{A \times D.F. \times 1000}{\xi \times d \times Hb\ (g/L)}$$

ξ: Extinction coefficient = 13.600 mM.$^{-1}$ cm^{-1}

D.F.: Dilution factor =137.5

d: light path = 1 cm

2.9.21. Erythrocyte glutathione peroxidase (GPx) assay:

Glutathione peroxidase was assayed according to the procedure of Paglia and Valantine [195] with some modifications of Pleban and Muny, [196] the recycling procedure for the determination of GPx activity depends on the oxidation of GSH to GSSG by the enzyme in the presence of NADPH and exogenous glutathione reductase which re-generates GSH from GSSG. The rate of enzyme activity is monitored by following the decrease in absorbance at 340 nm and 25°C as a function of NADPH exhaustion.

A) Reagents:

1) Double strength Drabkin's reagent.

2) GSH 92 mg in 10ml D.W. (freshly prepared).

3) NADPH 25µg in 10ml D.W. (freshly prepared).

4) NaN3: 39 mg in 10ml D.W.

5) GRx (Type III) 0.5mg in 10 ml Phosphate buffer.

6) Phosphate buffer, 0.15M, PH 7.0 contains 0.005M EDTA.

7) H_2O_2 80 µl of 30% solution in 100 ml D.W. Prepare immediately before assay.

B) Hemolysate preparation:

1) 0.1ml of packed cell volume was transferred to 0.4ml D.W., and freezed overnight.

2) After thawing of hemolysate, the hemolysate was centrifuged to remove cell depress.

3) 0.1ml of supernatant was added to a tube contains 1.9ml D.W. and mixed.

4) 1.0 ml of this solution was combined with 1.0 ml double-strength Drabkin's regents, and then leaved for 20min.

C) Assay:

Reagent	Test(ml)	Blank(ml)
1. Phosphate buffer	1.0	1.0
2. H_2O	1.4	1.5
3. GSH	0.1	0.1
4. GRx	0.1	0.1
5. NaN_3	0.1	0.1
6. NADPH	0.1	0.1
7. Hemolysate	0.1	----
8. H_2O_2	0.1	0.1
Final Volume	3.0	3.0

The reaction was initiated by the addition of H_2O_2 to the assay mixture and change in absorbance was monitored for 10 min period of time at 340nm and 25°C. Hemoglobin concentration was determined for the solution in step (2) of hemolysate preparation.

D) Calculation:

Calculation was made with the use of molar extinction coefficient 6.22 mM.$^{-1}$cm^{-1} for NADPH, and enzyme activity was determined from the following formula.

$$GPx\ activity\ in\ RBC\ (U/g\ Hb) = \frac{\dfrac{\Delta A}{t} \times V_t \times 1000}{\xi \times V_s \times d \times Hb(g/L)}$$

ΔA: Difference in absorbance

V_t: Total volume of assay = 3.0 ml

V_s: sample volume = 0.1 ml

ξ: Extinction coefficient = 6.22 mM.$^{-1}$ cm^{-1}

d: Length of light path = 1.0 cm

Hb: Hemoglobin concentration in hemolysate.

t: time interval (10 min).

2.9.22. Erythrocyte glutathione reductase (GRx) assay:

Glutathione reductase activity was determined by the method of West [197] with minor modifications from Lee [198]. The enzyme catalyzes the reduction of glutathione disulfide GSSG) to the corresponding reduced from (GSH), and the reaction proceeds by the presence of NADPH. The enzyme activity can be measured by monitoring the decrease in absorbance at 340 nm and 37°C.

A) Reagents:

1) Potassium phosphate buffer 0.1 M, pH 7.4.

2) EDTA, 1.4889g in 100ml D.W.

3) NADPH 25 µg in 10ml D.W. (Freshly).

4) GSSG 0.1 l0gm in 10ml D.W. (freshly).

B) Hemolysate Preparation:

1) 0.lml of packed cell volume was added to 0.4 ml D.W. and then stored at (-20°C) overnight.

2) After thawing, the hemolysate was centrifuged to remove the stoma.

3) 0.lml of supernatant was added to1.9 ml D.W. and vortex well.

4) 0.5 ml of hemolysate was assayed in step (3) for Hb determination.

C) Assay:

Reagents	Test(ml)	Blank(ml)
1. Buffer	2.6	2.6
2. Hemolysate	0.1	---
3. EDTA	0.1	0.1
4. GSSG	0.1	0.1
5.H_2O	---	0.1
6. NADPH	0.1	0.1
Final Volume	3.0	3.0

The reaction was started by the addition of NADPH, and the change in absorbance was monitored at 37°C and 340nm wavelength for 10 min time interval.

E) Calculation:

$$GRx \text{ activity in RBC (U/g Hb)} = \frac{\frac{\Delta A}{t} \times V_t \times 1000}{\xi \times V_s \times d \times Hb(g/L)}$$

ΔA: Difference in absorbance

V_t : Total volume of assay = 3.0 ml

Vs: sample volume =0.1 ml

ξ : Extinction coefficient = 6.22 mM.$^{-1}$ cm $^{-1}$

d: Length of light path = 1.0 cm

Hb: Hemoglobin concentration in hemolysate.

t: time interval (10 min).

$$GR_x \text{ activity in RBC (U/g Hb)} = \frac{48.23 \times \Delta A}{Hb \ (g/dl)}$$

2.9.23. Determination of erythrocyte catalase activity (CAT) [199]

Procedure:

1- Hemolysate by using RBC: D.W. (1:4, v/v) was prepared.

2- 20 µl of hemolysate was diluted with 10 ml phosphate buffer.

3- 1ml buffer plus 2 ml diluted hemolysate were mixed in Blank tube.

4- 2ml of diluted hemolysate was added to 1 ml of hydrogen peroxide solution, mixed well and absorbance was measured immediately at 240 nm. Then the absorbance was measured after 15 sec.

Calculation:

$$K = (2.303 / \Delta_t) \times \log A_1/A_2 \times 60$$

A_1 = Absorbance at time (zero) and A_2 = Absorbance at time (15 sec)

2.9.24. Determination of erythrocyte superoxide dismutase (SOD) activity:

Superoxide dismutase activity in erythrocyte was determined by using a modified photochemical nitro-blue tetrazolium (NBT) method utilizing sodium cyanide as peroxidase inhibitor [200].

Reagents:

(1)-Working phosphate buffer 50 mM (pH 7.8) containing 0.1 mM EDTA and triton x-100(0.025%) This solution was prepared as follows:

Solution A: Dipotassium hydrogen orthophosphate (50 mM).Dissolve 8.709 gm of Dipotassium hydrogen orthophosphate in about 250 ml deionized water and then the total volume is completed to 1 liter.

Solution B: potassium dihydrogen orthophosphate (50mM).Dissolve 6.805 gm of potassium dihydrogen orthophosphate in about 250 ml of deionized water, then the total volume is completed to 1 liter.

Then mix 800 ml of solution A and 200 ml of solution B , adjust the pH to 7.8..The working buffer solution is prepared by adding 0.0375 gm EDTA and 0.25 ml of triton x-100 in phosphate buffer(50 mM) pH7.8 and the total volume is completed up to 1 liter with phosphate buffer.

(2) L-Methonine solution (0.2M): Dissolve 0.3 gm of L-Methonine in 10 ml of D.W.

(3) NBT-2HCL solution (1 .73 mM): Dissolve 0.0141 gm of NBT-2HCL in 10 ml .water.

.(4) Triton x-100 (1 %W/V) in D.W.

(5) Riboflavin solution (117 mM): Dissolve 0.0011 gm of riboflavin in 25 ml of .D.W

(6) Sodium cyanide solution (2mM).Dissolve 0.011 gm of sodium cyanide in 10 ml of D. H_2O

(7) Reacting mixture solution (Beyer et al 1987).This solution is prepared by mixing the following reagents. Reagent 1(17ml), Reagent 2(1.5ml), Reagent3 (1 ml), Reagent 4 (0.75ml).

Procedure:

(1) After preparation hemolysate solution add in dry test tubes as in the protocol assay below:

Solution No.	Blank Tube	Test tube
Working mixture solution	2.0 ml	2.0 ml
Sodium Azide solution	0.1 ml	0.1 ml
Hemolysate solution	---	0.1 ml
D.W.	0.86 ml	0.76 ml
Riboflavin solution	0.04ml	0.04 ml

(2) The contents of all tubes were mixed well and then measured the absorbance immediately at 560 nm.

(3) All tubes were illuminated by two fluorescent lamps (20 watt each) incubated in an aluminum foil lined box at 25 C for 10 minutes (75×50×20) cm . The intensity of incident light (I_o at 10 minutes is equal to 5,596x10 Einstein /sec.

(4) A inhibition calibration curve was made using normal erythrocyte cells at different volumes (20, 40, 60, 80, 100, 120, 160, 200, 240, and 260 µl) as shown in figure (2-3), and the % inhibition calculated as follows: The enzymatic activity of SOD is determined in reference to the difference in

optical density (O.D) before and after illumination comparison with control tube.

$$\% \text{ INHIBITION} = (\Delta B) - (\Delta T) / (\Delta B) \times 100$$

ΔB= Absorbance of blank after illumination - Absorbance of blank before illumination.

ΔT= Absorbance of Test after illumination - Absorbance of Test before illumination.

SOD Unit = 1/2 Inhibition = 37 % from the standard inhibition curve so,

SOD activity (U) = Inhibition of Test / 37 %

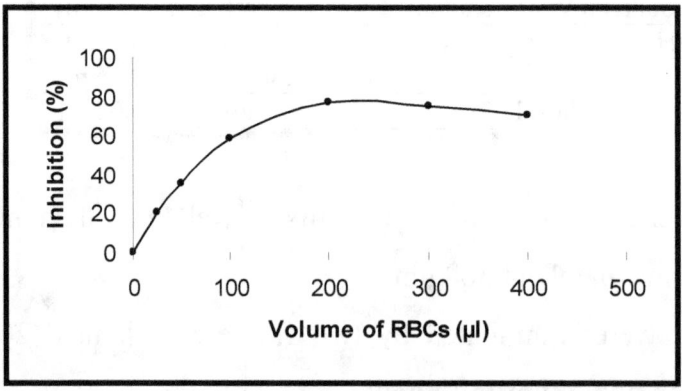

Figure 2-3. Calibration curve of SOD determination.

2.9.25. Determination of serum vitamin E by RP-HPLC:

A method by Bieri [201] was used to determine serum α-tocopherol by RP-HPLC with ultraviolet detection at 280 nm. Separation of α-tocopherol was carried out using a Nova-pak C18 stainless steel column (3.9 x 150 mm).The guard column was packed with the same material. The mobile phase used was methanol. Tocopherol acetate was used as internal standard. The injection volume was 50 μl, and the flow rate was 2 ml/min at room temperature. Serum α- tocopherol   was extracted with hexane.

2.9.26. Determination of serum vitamin C:

Serum vitamin C was measured colorimetrically according to the method of Lin [202] using a commercially available kit (Randox .England).

Procedure:

Material	AsA oxidase (treated tube)	Free tube
Test or standard	0.2 ml	0.2 ml
Ascorbic acid oxidase (working solution)	0.1 ml	------
Distill water	-----	0.1 ml
Mix. Well and incubate at 37C in water bath for 15 minutes. Then add as follows:		
Acetate buffer pH= 3.6	2.5 ml	2.5 ml
TPTZ solution	0.3 ml	0.3 ml
FeCl₃ solution	0.2 ml	0.2 ml

Gently mix the contents of each tube after each addition and allow standing at room temperature for exactly 5 min and reading spectrophotometrically at 593 nm.

2.9.27. Determination of serum β-carotene levels by HPLC:

The method of Bieri [203] was used to determine serum β-carotene using RP-HPLC with visible detection at 435 nm and peak automatic integration. Separation of β-carotene was carried out using a Nova-pak C18 (5μm) stainless steel column (3.9 ×150 mm. I'd).The guard column was packed with the same material. The mobile phase used was acetonitril/ dichloeoethane/ methanol (70:20:10). The injection volume was 60μl and flow rate was 1 ml/ min at room temperature. Plasma carotene was extracted with hexane (0.025% BHT).

2.9. 28. Determination of serum total antioxidant capacity:

The spectrophotometric method by Rice–Evan [204] was performed to measure the total antioxidant capacity of the sample using a commercially available kit (Randox, England). ABTS is incubated with myoglobin and hydrogen peroxide to produce the cation radical. The ABTS$^+$ radical generate a relatively stable blue-green stain which is measured at 600 nm. The antioxidants in serum reduce the intensity of staining in proportion to their total content. A cuvette needs to be prepared for each of the following solutions:

Blank reagent: 20 μl of water and 1 ml of chromogen solution; Standard: 20 μl of standard and 1 ml of chromogen solution; and Sample: 20 μl of plasma and 1 ml of chromogen solution. The tubes were mixed well and then the absorbance was measured(A_1), 200 μl of hydrogen peroxide was added to all solutions, mixed well again and then leaved for 3 min; the absorbance was measured again (A_2). The absorbance values obtained yield the total antioxidant capacity, expressed in μmol/l of Trolox, by the following formulae:

$$A_{2sample} - A_{1sample} = \Delta A\ sample$$
$$A_{2standard} - A_{1standard} = \Delta A\ standard$$
$$A_{2blank} - A_{1blank} = \Delta A\ blank$$
$$F = standard\ /\ (A_{blank} - A_{standard})$$
$$Antioxidant\ capacity\ (\mu mol/L) = F \times (A_{Blank} - A_{sample})$$

2.10. Microbiologic studies

2.10.1 *Organism*s:

Five standard strains supplied from Central health Laboratary used in this study *Staphylococcus aureus* ATCC 25923, *Klebsiella pneumonia* ATCC 3600, *E.coli* ATCC 6750. *H.influenza* ATCC 9006. *Salmonella typhi* ATCC 7445.On the other hand ten fresh clinical isolates obtained from patients attending central health Laboratary were identified morphologically by strain biochemical testing .These clinical isolates included, (*Salmonella typhi* 2 strains, *Staphylococcus aureus* 2 stains, *E.coli* 2 strains, *Klebseilla Pneumonia* 2 strains , *and H. influenza* 2 strain , causal agents of intestinal, respiratory tract and urinary tract infections in man were tested for *in vitro* susceptibility of oleuropein.

2.10.2. *Oleuropein sensitivity Test*:

Bacterial strains were tested for their susceptibility to antimicrobial activity of phenolic compounds (oleuropein, oleuropein aglycone, hydroxytyrosol, and elenolic acid) by paper disc method described by the Bauer [205].

A Mueller–Hinton agar was used for this purpose. When sterilized medium comes to 45-50 C, it was poured into Petri dishes, Agar depth must be 4mm. For 90 mm diameter plates 25 ml medium was enough, pH of the medium must be 7.2-7.4., then from primary isolation medium 4-5 colonies that show similar morphology were taken by flamed loop and suspended in 4-5 ml broth(Mueller-Hinton; Trypticase soy broth or brain heart infusion). They were incubated in 37 C for 2-5 hours. If a viable turbidity was obtained at the end of this period, the turbidity of bacterial suspension was adjusted against Mac Farland Standard Tube (0.5 ml 1.175% $BaCl_2.2H_2O$ solution + 99.5 ml 0.36N (1%) H_2SO_4 solution) with physiologic serum or broth and inoculation was performed. If the concentration of bacteria was small, inoculation was done after 2-8 hours from incubation. The inoculation into Petri dishes had been doing according to the technique reported by Bauer and Kirby [205]

Prepared bacterial suspension was mixed with sterile applicator and excess fluid of applicator was removed by rotating the applicator to one side of the tube. The applicator was streaked on the entire agar surface in three different directions by rotating the plates at 60 C angles after each striking. The applicator must be rubbed to the whole surface of the plate.

Afterwards, Petri dishes allowed drying for 15-20 minutes at room temperature, then, cartridge was opened under flame, and then discs were discharged from cartridge onto the Petri dish by means of trigger. It was necessary to press gently on the dispersed discs by the help of a flamed and cooled forceps. To see inhibition zone clearly, the space between discs must not be narrower than 24 mm and the distance of discs from the edges of the plate must be one cm.

Inoculated Petri dishes must be put into incubator in inverse position, after incubation at 37 C for one night, the zones occurred must be evaluated according to the authentic minimum inhibition diameters [206]. Accordingly, the results were evaluated as susceptible, intermediate and resistant respectively.

2.10.3. Determination of MIC and MBC of oleuropein on different species of bacteria:

Susceptibility tests were performed on each bacterial strain using the tube dilution technique [206]. A series dilutions in Mueller-Hinton broth of the phenolic compounds listed above were prepared (using overnight broth culture diluted 1:1000 to give 10^5 colony forming unit (CFU/ml).The series dilution were contained a concentration (320, 160, 80, 40, 20, 10, 5, 2.5, 1.25 µg/ml of each oleuropein and its related metabolites, oleuropein aglycone, hydroxytyrosol and elenolic acid). To a sterile tube which contains each series of concentration as mentioned above add 1 ml of a bacterial suspension (10^5CFU/ml) against tube without phenolic compound used as a control. Then all tubes were incubated at 37 C for 24 hours. Results were read after 24 h and the MIC, where no growth appeared, was determined for each bacterial strain under study.

The minimum bactericidal concentration (MBC) was determined by taking 100 µl of inoculated tubes which have no growth turbidity and inoculated on a nutrient agar, incubated for 24 hours at 37C. Any Petri dishes have no growth considered a MBC [207].

2.11. Radioreceptor assay studies

2.11.1. Isolation of lymphocytes cells and binding experiments with labeled insulin:

For isolation lymphocytes, blood was collected from healthy and NIDDM patients. The lymphocyte cells were isolated by centrifugation through lymphoprep and washed free of protein as previously reported by Al-Azzawie 1986 [208]. Viability of the cells was monitored by trypan blue dye exclusion. Hundred-million lymphocytes were incubated with increasing concentrations of I^{125}-insulin (initial specific activity of insulin labeled (500μci/μg) with or without addition of unlabelled insulin. Incubation was carried out in a protein free medium (Eagle's Medium) at different temperatures 15, 25, 37, 45 °C for 10-90 min. Specific insulin binding was determined by removing aliquots onto chilled buffer in plastic micro tubes and centrifuged as previously described by Gaven [209] .Using the 15 C° incubation, we observed no loss of viability in the cell suspensions or decrease in binding even at high densities of peripheral lymphocytes. In contrast to similar incubations at higher temperatures allowed more accurate measurements of the binding kinetic of the insulin -lymphocyte interaction.

2.12.2. Determination of DNA. [210]

A method of Burton 1956 was carried out to measuring the a mount of DNA in lymphocyte cells .When DNA treated with diphenylamine under acidic conditions a blue compound was formed with a sharp absorption maxima at 595 nm.

Reagents:

1- Diphenylamine reagent was prepared by dissolving 1.50 gm of diphenylamine in 100 ml glacial acetic acid, and then the reagent kept well at dark place.

2- Acetaldehyde solution was prepared by taking 0.20 ml of acetaldehyde completed to 10 ml by distilled water.0.1 ml from this solution was used with 20 ml of diphenylamine.

3- Standard DNA solution was prepared by dissolving 50 mg from calf thymus DNA in 100 ml of 0.5 N perchloric acid. The solution was heated until 75 C for 30 min, and then kept at 4 C.

4- Perchloric acid solution prepared by diluting 50 ml of 20%perchloric acid to 200 ml with distilled water.

Assay

The reagents were added in the tubes as in the following diagram, and then mixed well, Boiled at 100 C for 10 minutes, Cooled and the absorbance at 600 nm was measured and DNA concentration was calculated after calibration curve of standard DNA.

Reagent*	B.tube	Standard Tube				T.tube
	1	2	3	4	5	6
Standard DNA solution (50mg/dl)	-----	0.1	0.2	0.4	0.8	-----
Suspension of lymphocyte cells	-----	-----	-----	-----	-----	0.5
Perchloric acid solution (0.5N)	1	0.9	0.8	0.6	0.2	0.5
Diphenylamine solution	2	2l	2	2	2	2

* All values are given as ml.

2.11.3. Calculation

1. The B/T % ratio was computed for each tube, where B is the bound radioactivity mean counts (cpm) which represents the (l^{125}-insulin binding to lymphocyte cell). F is the free radioactivity mean counts which represents the non-bound l^{125}-insulin, while T is the total radioactivity mean of the counts of l^{125}-insulin, so F = T - B

2. The concentration of the Bound in fmol/100 µg DNA that formed after time (t) was calculated from the following equation:

B = fmol/100 µg DNA =B (cpm) / T (cpm) x conc. I^{125}-insulin used in the incubation medium.

3. The affinity constant and maximal binding capacity was determined according to Scatchard equation.

$$B/F = K_a \, B - B_{max}$$

K_a = Affinity constant,

K_d = Dissociation constant

B_{max} = Maximal binding capacity.

Since MBC / number of lymphocyte cells used = number of binding sites per one lymphocyte cell (number of receptors).

4. The values of the ratio B/F were plotted against the values of the (B) in fmol/100 µg DNA give a curvilinear relationship. The values of each affinity constant at each temperature can be calculated from the slope of the straight line, while the value of the total concentration of binding sites (B_{max}) was calculated from the intercept with the x-axis.

2.12. Histological Studies:

2.12.1 Animals used

Swiss albino mice of the balb/c strain were used in this study, the mice were in good health 2-3 months of age, weighing between 25-30 gm of both sex male and female, they were breed in the animal house in the college of agriculture and kept in plastic cages. The animals were kept in a room temperature.

2.12.2. Experimental Design

The experiment was carried on eighteen mice were divided into three groups, each group contained 6 mice of both male and female, each group was separated in three cages, two cages contained male mice and the other cage contained female mice in order to avoid accidental pregnancy.

Group (1): The first group were the healthy, they were given (200 μl) soy oil

Group (2): The second group of animals were injected intraperitonealy with a dose of 150 mg/kg alloxan, in order to prevent severe hypoglycemia, alloxan treated animals received a solution of 10 % glucose, instead of normal drinking water over the 24 hours following the treatment with alloxan as reported by Cignarella [211].

Group (3): The third group of animals was experimentally treated with a dose of 150 mg/kg alloxan in addition to orally given the pure oleuropein isolated and purified as shown previously in page (66) at a dose of 100 mg/kg everyday for three weeks in 200 μl of soy oil.

2.12.3. Sampling

Animals were anaesthetized by diethyl ether and then scarified at dated 1, 2, and 3 weeks of the experiment, beginning with the control group. The abdominal cavity was opened and small pieces of the pancreas were taken for light microscopic preparations.

2.12.4. Histological Technique

A-Fixation procedure

Tissue specimens used for light microscopic histological investigation were fixed in Boun solution for 24 hours as reported by Bancroft [212] .The fixative was prepared as follow: Saturated aqueous of picric acid solution (75 ml) was dissolved in 25 ml of 40% formaldehyde then 5 ml of glacial acetic acid was added to the solution.

B- Tissue preparation

After fixation, the specimen were dehydrated by series of ethanol alcohol, cleared in xylene then impregnated and embedded in paraffin wax in an oven for 4-6 hr, and then the specimens were blocked in paraffin wax. Serial transverse of 4-5 µ thickness were cut by using the microtome, the sections then floated in a water bath at 50C, and mounted on a slide by using Mayer's albumin, then passed through special staining methods as reported by Bancroft [212].

The diameter average of islets of Langerhans studied (longitudinal and horizontal diameter for each islets) at the first, second and third week in ten sections for each animal by selecting each 3rd section randomly as reported by Al-Shaikh [213].

C- Staining methods

Orange Fuchin Green method (O.F.G)

This method has been described by Slidders [214]. It has been chosen because it is used in the staining of islets of Langerhans.

1- Section of 4 micron thickness, mounted on slide were dewaxed in xylene then rehydrated by 100%, 95%,70% EtOH for 2-3 minutes for each , then in running water.

2- The nuclei were stained for 3 minutes by Celestin Blue Haemalum.

3- Washed twice with tap water.

4- Stained with Mayer Hematoxylin for 5 minutes.

5- Washed with tap water.

6- Differentiated in 0.25% HCL which is dissolved in 70 % EtOH.

7- Washed with tap water.

8- Washed with 95% EtOH for 3-5 min.

9- Stained with a saturated solution of 0.5% of orange-G-Stain

10- Washed with tap water.

11-Stained with a solution of Acid Fuchsin 0.5% dissolved in acetic acid (0.5% for 3-5 min).

12- Washed with distill water.

13- Cleared with a solution of 1 % phosphotungestic acid.

14 -Washed with D.W.

15-Stained with a solution of 2% Light Green stain dissolved in 1.5% acetic acid.

16-Rinsed with distill water to remove the remaining stains.

17-Washed with absolute alcohol for 1-2 min.

extracts, the oleuropein content and solids content can be determined. Then, the contents can be adjusted so that the correct oleuropein content is obtained in the powder after drying, preferably 30% by weight. The oleuropein obtained by the method of the extraction can be administered orally and oral dosage forms can be in a solid or liquid form. Such dosage forms can be formulated from purified oleuropein or they can be formulated from aqueous or aqueous-alcoholic extracts. Regarding the latter, aqueous or aqueous-alcoholic (e.g., water-methanol or water-ethanol) extracts can be spray dried to provide a dry powder that can be formulated into oral dosage forms with other pharmaceutically acceptable carrier.

3.1.1. Total phenolic compounds content and antioxidant activity in olive leaves extract.

Potential sources of antioxidant compounds have been searched from several types of plant material by using a number of different methods. Flavonoids and other phenolic are especially common in leaves. The antioxidant activity of phenolic is mainly due to their redox properties which allow them to act as reducing agents, hydrogen donors and singlet oxygen quenchers [215]. The purpose of this study was to screen the total phenolic compounds content and antioxidant activity of different extracts made from three variety of *olea europeae* cultivated in Iraq. The Labeeb, Al-Asharsy and Manzanillo were the materials of interest.

The Folin-Ciocalteu colorimetric assay applied in this study is a simple method and requires few reagents, thus being suitable for crude estimation of the content of total phenols, even though it is limited by the low specificity toward polyphenols and relies on the use of a standard compound [216].The highest total phenolic content was occurred in the extracts of Labeeb then Al-asharsy and finally Manzanillo type. The results obtained in the determination of total phenolic and the test of antioxidant activity were used as a basis for selecting the type of olive leaves extract used in further studies for determination its biological activity as shown from table (3-2).

Table 3-2. Total phenolic compounds as gallic acid equivalent (GAE) in different varieties of olive leaf extracts (Mean ± SD µg/ml).

Variety of Olive Tree	n	T. phenolic (GAE)
Labeeb	4	333 ±3.4
Al-Asharsy	4	226 ± 4.2
Manzanillo	4	180 ± 3.7
Bid el Hamman (control)	2	165 ± 3.5

3.1.2. Rapid HPLC method for determination oleuropein in olive leaves extract:

Chromatographic profiles of the different *olea europeae* varieties studied showed non differences in qualitative composition. The main compounds detected by HPLC as shown in figure (3-1a, b, c,) were identified as rutin (Retention time = 6.8 min), verbascoside (7.8 min), luteolin 7-glucoside (9 min), apigenin 7-glucoside (15.3 min), and oleuropein 23.5 min and oleuroside (33.8 min). The unidentified compound (16.5 min is currently under investigation). Its UV spectrum suggests a flavonoids structure Demethyloleuropein was not detected in leaf extracts of the three varieties studied, ("Labeeb, Al-asharsy and Manzanillo) when compared with the Bid el Haman variety which used as control (Figure 3-1d).Oleuropein concentration in leaves was calculated in percentage (w/w) for each variety as shown in table (3-3) according to calibration curves which were plotted by correlating the area ratio(oleuropein/internal standard) versus the corresponding concentration ratios.

Samples were collected from three varieties and short sampling time (5 days) made seasonal variations irrelevant. The two Iraqi varieties had concentration of (14.50 ± 2.5, & 12.03 ± 2.2 mg/g) while the Manzanillo (Spanish variety had the lowest concentration (10.62 ± 1.9) mg/g dry weight of olive leaves. Values obtained in this study were higher than usually reported in relation to Manzanillo variety, in the drying method rather than the extraction method. A previous study by Ellias [217] showed that microwave drying avoid ester hydrolysis of saponion which occurred with air drying.

Table 3-3. Oleuropein concentration (mg/g dry weight of olive leaves) in four cultivated varieties of *Olea europaea.*

Variety of Olive Tree	n	Oleuropein conc.(mg/g)
Labeeb	4	14.50 ± 2.5
Al-Asharsy	4	12.03 ± 2.2
Manzanillo	4	10.62 ± 1.9
Bid el Hamman(control)	2	13.22 ± 1.2

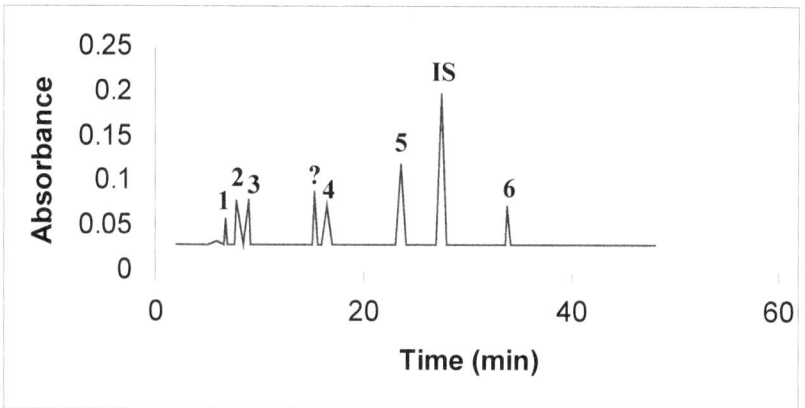

Figure 3-1 a. HPLC chromatogram of an extract of olea europaea from **Labeeb Variety**. Peak =1rutin; 2= verbascoside; 3= luteolin 7- glucoside; 4=apigenin 7-glucoside; 5= oleuropein; 6=oleuroside; I.S= Coumarin? = unknown compound. Detection was at 280 nm.

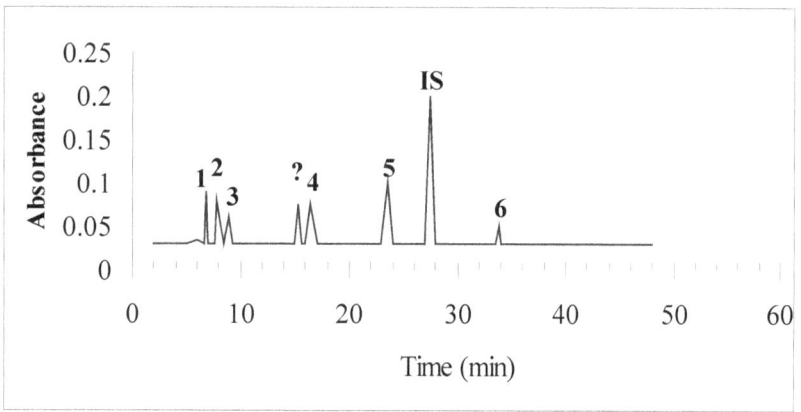

Figure 3-1 b. HPLC chromatogram of an extract of olea europaea leaves from **Al-asharsy variety**. Peak 1= rutin; 2= verbascoside; 3=Luteolin 7-glucoside; 4=apigenin 7-glucoside; 5= oleuropein; 6=oleuroside. I.S= coumarin? = unknown compound. Detection was at 280 nm.

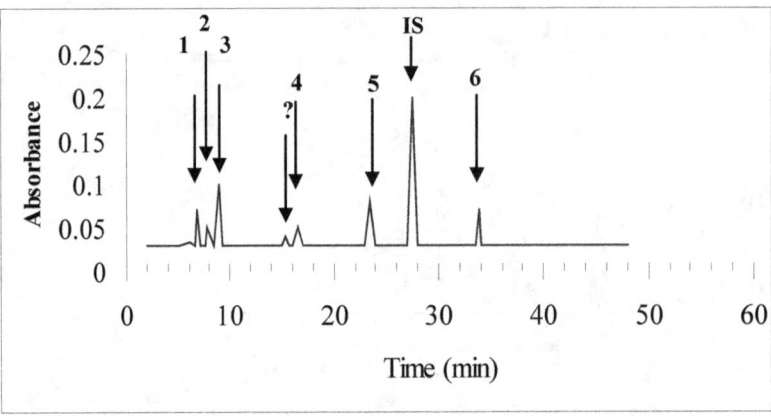

Figure 3-1 c. HPLC chromatogram of an extract of olea europeae leaves from **Manzanillo variety**. Peak 1= rutin; 2= verbascoside; 3= luteolin 7-glucoside; 4=apigenin 7-glucoside; 5= Oleuropein; 6= oleuroside; I.S. coumarin., ? = unknown compound. Detection at 280 nm.

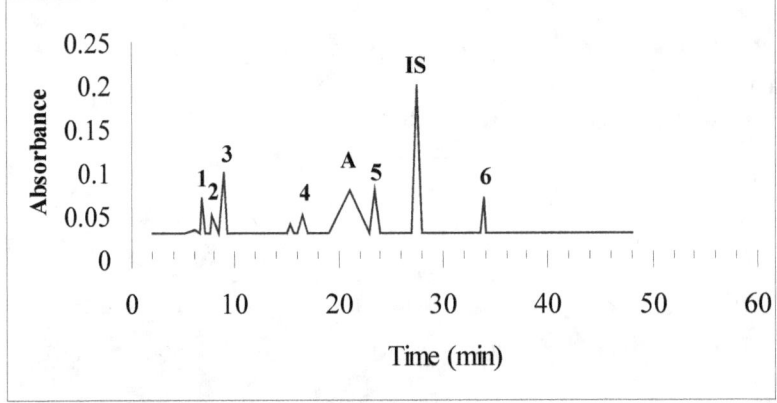

Figure 3-1 d. HPLC chromatogram of olea europaea leaves from **Bid el Haman variety (Control)**. Peak 1= rutin; 2= verbascoside; 3= luteolin 7-glucoside; 4=apigenin 7-glucoside; 5=oleuropein; 6= oleuroside; .I.S coumarin. Detection was at 280 nm. (Peak A= Demethyloleuropein)

The isocratic HPLC method described in this study allowed rapid separation and identification of the major compounds of olive leaves. The quantitation of oleuropein using an internal standard is of particular importance because commercially available oleuropein standards are not of HPLC grade. This method could be used for routine analysis of leaves, extracts and industrial products. The chromatographic profiles and the evaluation of compound, distribution, especially oleuropein could lead to characterization of varieties and evaluation of their homogeneity. In the varieties studied, the Iraqi al-asharsy and particularly labeeb had high oleuropein concentration. Studies of ecological and culture conditions should permit optimization of culture conditions for olive leaf crops.

Analyses of the HPLC spectra of extracts confirmed that the extract from Labeeb leaves possess the highest oleuropein content (14.50 ± 2.5 mg/ g dry weight) of powdered leaves, so it became the best candidate extraction. It is a well known fact that the phenolic compounds present in *Olea europaea* leaves vary in qualitative and quantitative terms, during the development and growth process, one of the main phenolic compounds is secoiridoid oleuropein, a heterosidic ester of glucosylated elenolic acid and 3,4-dihydroxy phenylethanol (hydroxytyrosol), responsible for bitterness in leaves, oil and olive fruits. Many molecules isolated from *Olea europaea* fruits and leaves are thought to have originated from oleuropein, via aglycone, by the opening of the elenolic acid ring with a final rearrangement into the secoiridoid compound, many forms of elenolic acid and simple phenolic compounds, such as hydroxytyrosol, moreover these molecules are known for their free radical scavenging activity, the biological effect of hydroxytyrosol has been explored in particular. Free radicals and their uncontrolled production, in fact, are responsible for several pathological processes, such as certain tumors (prostate and colon cancers) and coronary heart disease and diabetes.

3.1.3. Effect of solvent on the recovery of oleuropein in olive leaves extract

Methanol has been widely used for the extraction of phenolic compounds from a variety of matrices [218] and its use for olive leaf was examined in this study .The effect on selectivity of incorporating water in the extracting solvent was monitored by HPLC analysis using gradient 1. Profiles were generally similar but significant quantitative differences were observed as illustrated in figure (3-2). A solvent comprising methanol / water (v/v) provided maximum relative recovery of phenolic including two strong peaks eluting at 16.8 min and 22.2 min as shown in figure (3-2). Thus, methanol / water (v/v) was determined to be the best extracting solvent with respect to selectivity and extraction efficiency. Similarly, an extraction time of 240 min at 60 C gave optimum recovery as assessed by comparison of chromatographic peak heights. On the other hand, a simple hexane wash was efficient in removing lipoid materials without loss of phenols.

The phenolic fraction of olive leaves represents a complex mixture that is difficult to resolve without complex gradients and ternary mobile phases. All three gradients used in this study provided adequate separations although resolution of some critical "pairs" required use of the shallower gradient (gradient 3) at the expense of analysis time as shown in table (3-4).

Detection at 240 nm provided lower selectivity particularly as seen in the detection of a split peak at 15.0 min (This peak, which was not detected by either fluorescence or absorption at 280 nm, was present in control chromatograms but increased significantly in extracts treated with acid or base, particularly after 2 hour (Figure 3-4 b& e). The increase in this peak coincided with a decrease in oleuropein. The identity of this peak has not been confirmed but previous studies suggest that it is incompletely resolved elenolic acid and elenolic acid glucoside. Profiles of free phenolic recovered from olive leaf by aqueous methanol extraction were dominated by the oleuropein peak (Figure 3-3a: peak 16) which was present as a major component in the samples of olive leaf extract, and as shown in figure 3-2, the quantitatively most significant phenols were eluted at 16.8 and 22.2 min. Both verbascoside and the oleuroside eluted much later than the 16.8 min seen for this compound which exhibited an absorption maximum at 331 nm with a shoulder at 298 nm. Oleuropein is generally considered the most significant olive phenol used in experiments on acid / base hydrolysis. Stability of the control extract at room temperature was examined over 24 hour and there was no significant reduction in the oleuropein content over 2 hour but a 14.8% loss after 24 hour storage **(**Table 3-5). On the other hand, the level of some of the minor components decreased after 2 hour storage and thus extracts should generally be examined with minimal delay or stored at low temperature in the dark. This variation in stability of the various phenols is not surprising in view of their different antioxidant capacities. Decomposition (oxidation, hydrolysis) of glycosides that are generally later-eluting may enhance the content of simpler early-eluting phenols.

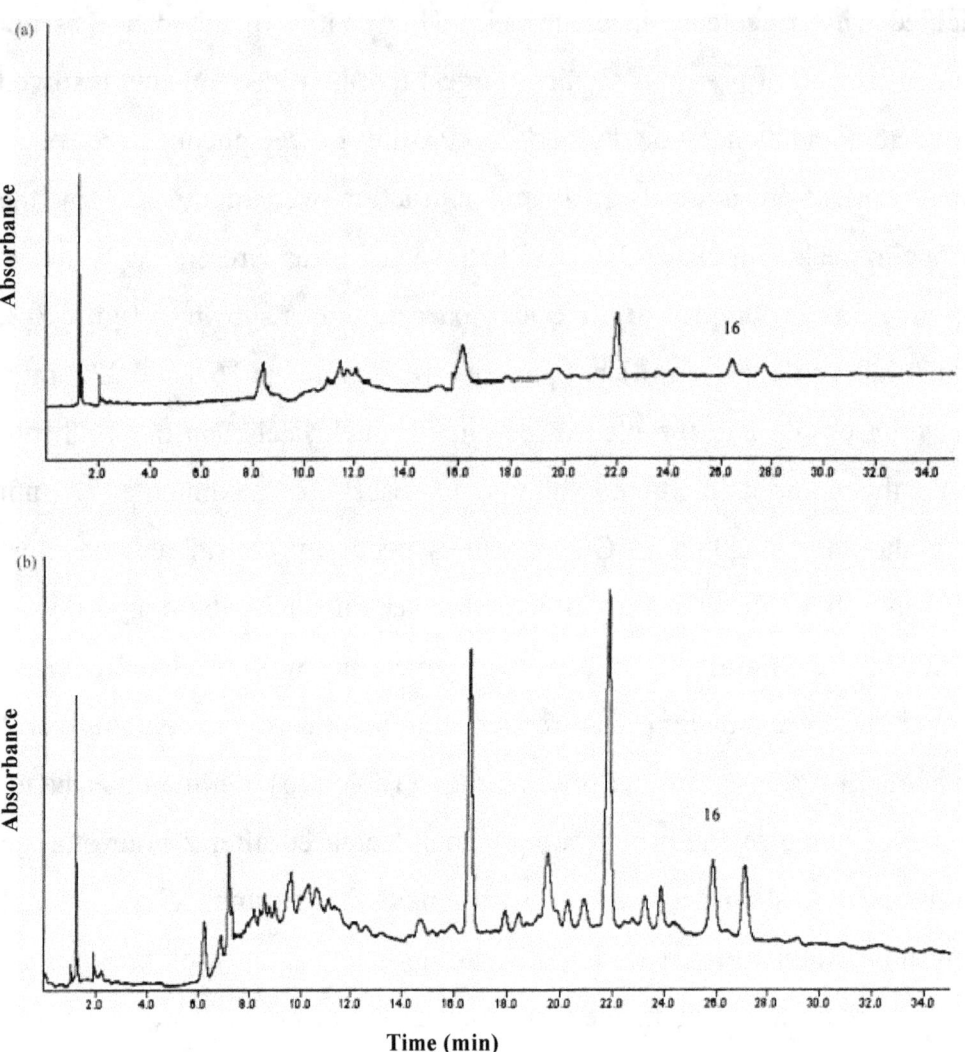

Figure 3-2. Chromatogram comparing the effect of different mixtures of aqueous methanol on extraction selectivity from olive leaves (Labeeb variety). Condition: gradient 1 with detection at 280 nm. Chromatograms are at fixed attenuation. Extracting solvents were **(a) methanol (100 % and (b) methanol + water (50 +50) v/v.**

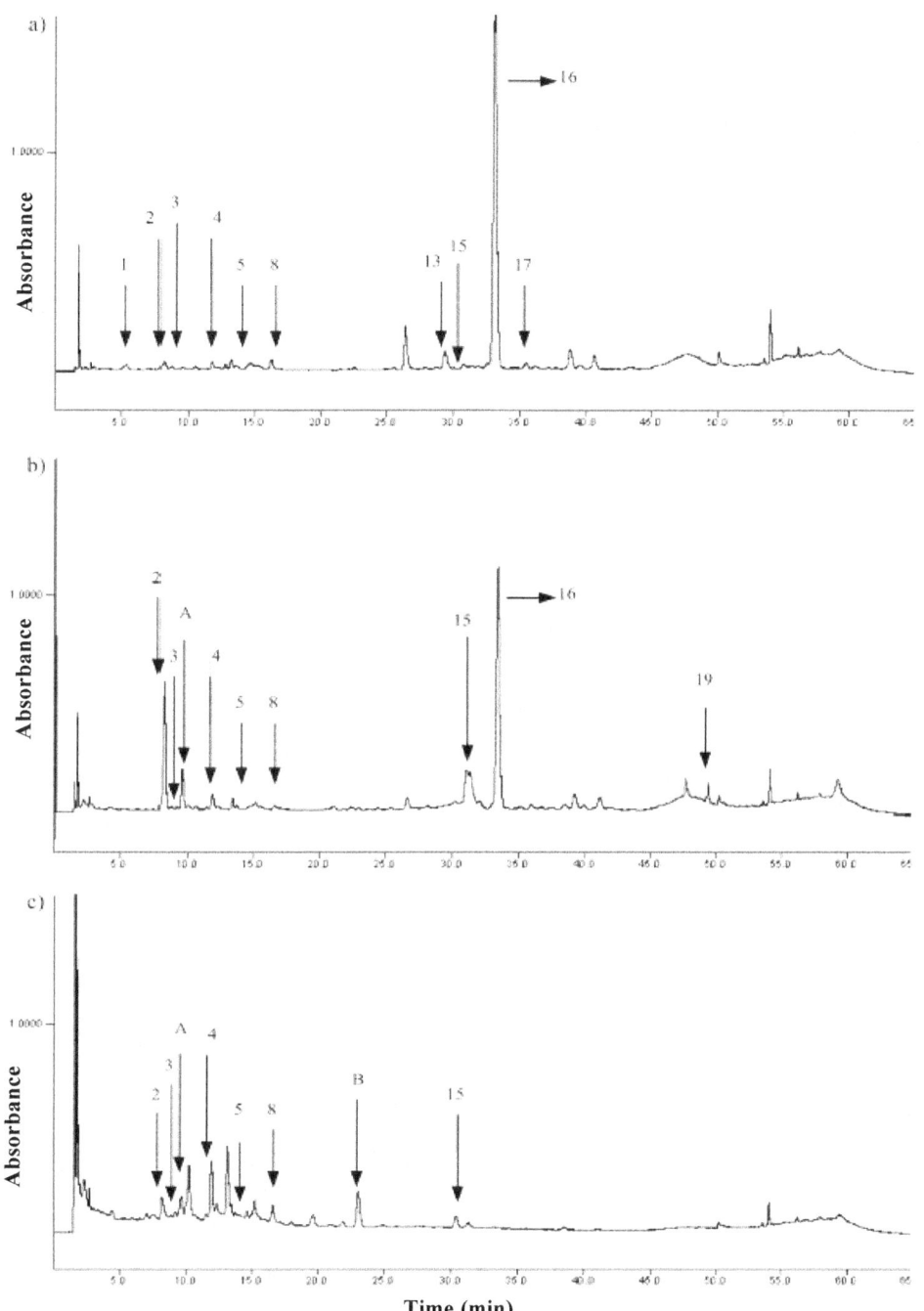

Figure 3-3. Chromatogram illustrating the effect of acid and base hydrolysis on the phenolic profile of olive leaves (Labeeb variety). Conditions: gradient 3 with detection at 280 nm. The different treatments were **(a) control: (b) acid hydrolysis for 2 hr, and (c) base hydrolysis for 2 hr**

Table 3-4. Retention time of selected mixture of standard phenolic compounds using gradient 3 carried out at the same conditions used in test samples.

Number	Phenolic Compound	Retention time (min)
1	Gallic acid	5.4
2	Hydroxytyrosol glucoside	8.2
3	Hydroxytyrosol	8.7
4	Tyrosol	11.8
5	Chlorogenic acid	14.6
6	Homovanillic acid	15
7	Vanillic acid	15.4
8	Caffeic acid	16.4
9	Syringic acid	16.6
10	P-Coumaric acid	22.7
11	Ferulic acid	24.4
12	Sinapic acid	24.8
13	O-Coumaric acid	29.7
14	Cyanidin chloride	29,9
15	Luteolin-7-glucoside	31
16	**Oleuropein**	33.3
17	Apeginin-7-glucoside	35.5
18	Luteolin	47
19	Apigenin	49

Table 3-5. The effect of acid and base extraction and hydrolysis on the concentrations of oleuropein in methanolic olive leaves extract. (Conc. in mg/g dried olive leaves).

Treatment	Time(h)	OH-tyrosol	Tyrosol	Caffeic acid	Oleuropein
	0	0.14	0.44	1.7	15.2
Control	2	0.13	0.12	0.65	15.1
	24	0.11	0.28	0.31	12.8
Acid extraction	2	1.4	0.38	0.30	6.33
	24	3.35	0.98	1.6	0.02
Acid hydrolysis	2	1.8	0.32	0.18	6.30
	24	3.7	0.94	1.5	0.02
Base extraction	2	0.4	1.3	1.3	0.05
	24	0.06	1.2	0.01	0.01
Base hydrolysis	2	0.57	1.5	0.95	0.04
	24	0.06	0.75	0.01	0.01

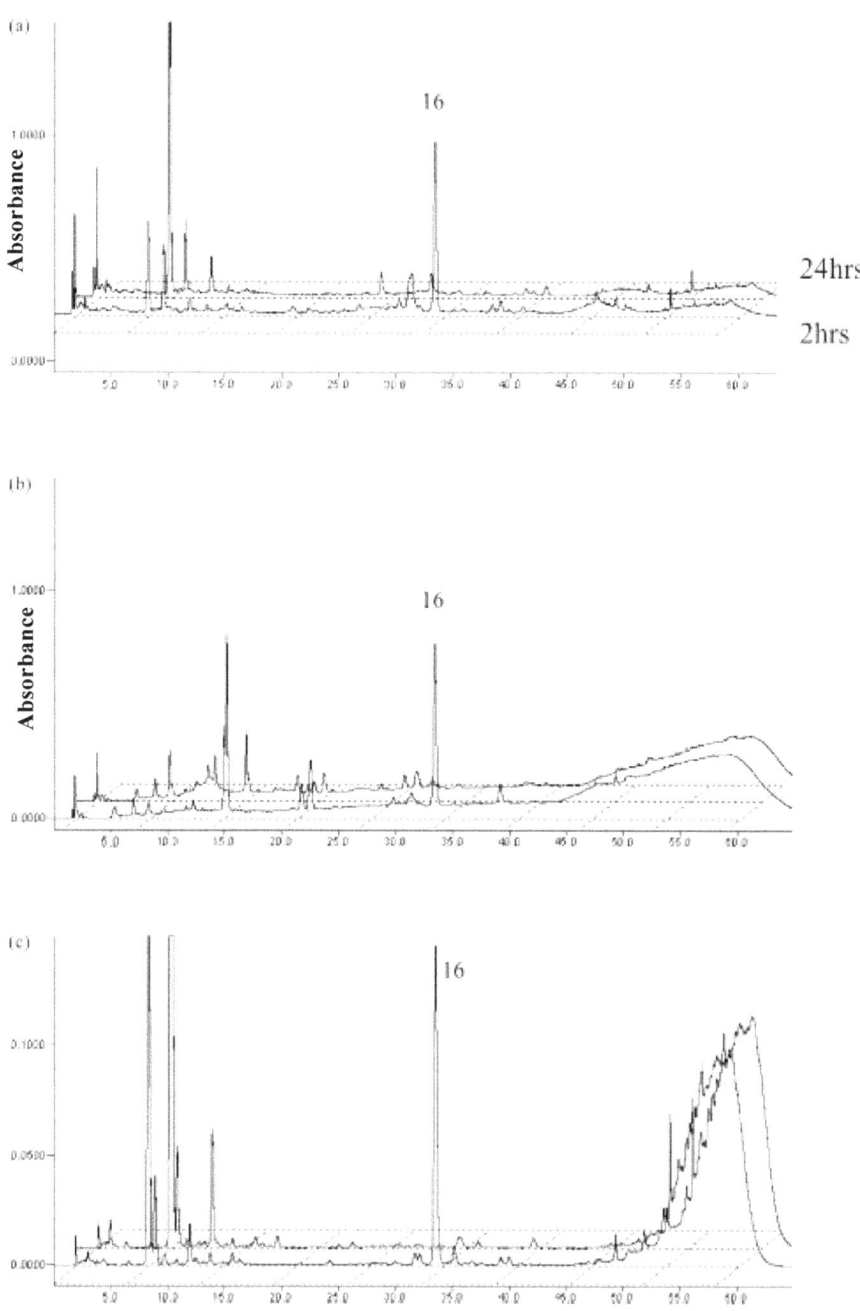

Figure 3-4. Chromatogram illustrating the effect of acid (a, b and c) and base (d, e and f) on phenolic profile of olive leaves(Labeeb variety) using different modes of detection as follows : (a) and (d) absorption at 280 nm; (b) and (e) absorption at 240 nm; and (c) and (f) fluorescence at 340 nm. The same intensity scales are used in (a), (b), (d) and (e) and in (c) and (f) {time in min}. In each case, the chromatogram in the foreground is shown after 24 hr treatment and that in the rear at 24 hour.

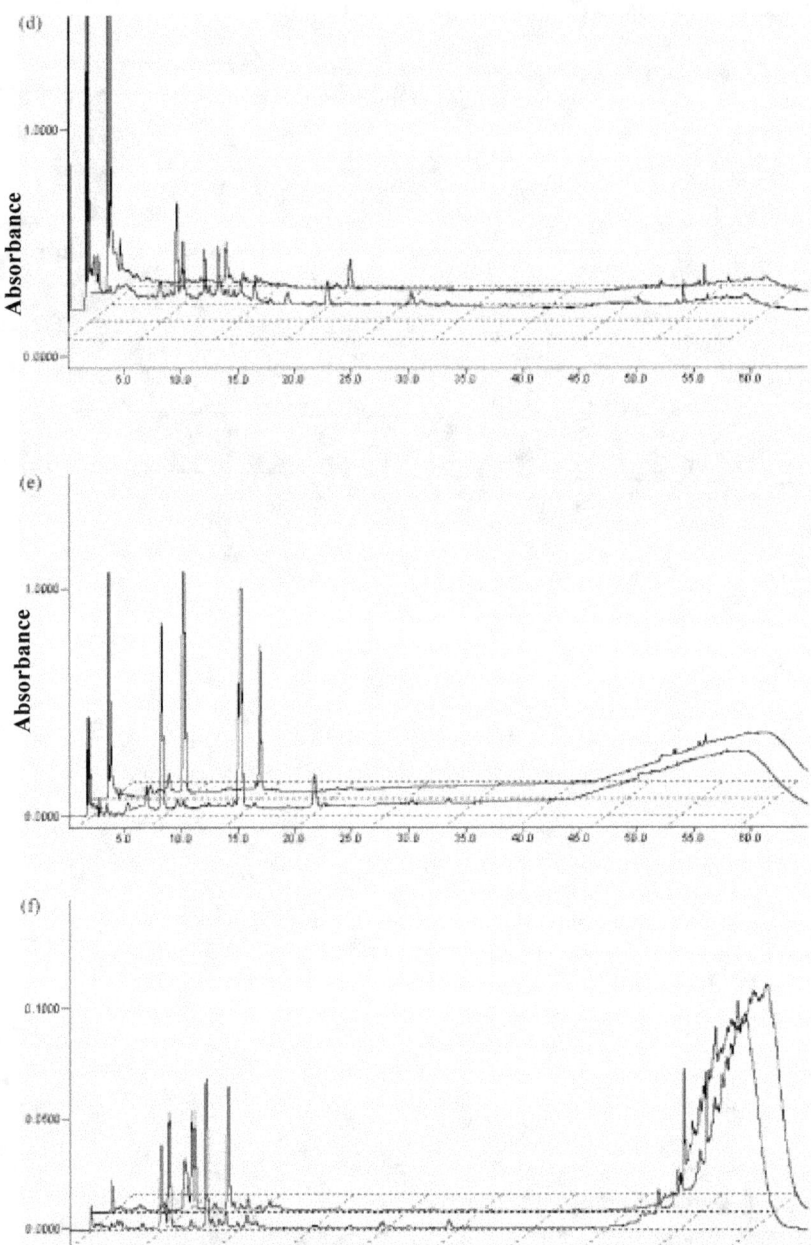

Time (min)

Figure 3-4. Continued

3.1.4. Effects of acid and base treatment on recovery of oleuropein in olive leaf extracts

Acid and base treatment of the aqueous methanol-extractable fraction induced hydrolysis or breakdown of the more complex, later-eluting phenolic species and enhanced the number and size of the early-eluting peaks (Figures 3-3 and 3-4). The most notable effect seen in the UV (240 and 280 nm absorption) and fluorescence chromatograms (280 nm excitation, 340 nm emission), was the reduction in the amount of oleuropein in both acid and base treated extracts. Acid-treatment (extraction and hydrolysis) produced a 40 and 99% loss in oleuropein after 2 and 24 hour, respectively. The corresponding values for base treatment (extraction and hydrolysis) were 98 and 100%, respectively. Caffeic acid is of particular interest as it is one of the major phenolic acids in plants, the level of caffeic acid in control samples decreased significantly after 2 hour, consistent with the reactivity of caffeic acid referred by its O-diphenolic grouping. However, the rise in level of caffeic acid at 24 hour can be attributed to degradation of caffeic containing species. In contrast, the addition of base to olive extracts resulted in an increase in caffeic acid concentration after 2 hour (compared to control extracts at 2 hour), followed by a complete disappearance after 24 hour. The levels of caffeic acid in acid treated extracts were more variable (Table 3-5).

Another significant difference between acid and base treatment of extracts was noticed in the formation of an unknown compound B (retention time 22.9 min) in base treated extracts (Figure 3-3c).The levels of this compound were very similar in base treated extracts after 2 and 24 hour. A further unknown compound A with retention time 9.6 min was produced in both acid and base treated extracts (Figure 3-3 b).

The amount of hydroxytyrosol produced was minimal although higher in base treated than acid treated extracts. Tyrosol was detected in acid and base treated extracts, but was higher in the latter. The origin of this is unclear but it may arise from ligstroside. The major degradation product from oleuropein in both acid and base treated extracts was hydroxytyrosol. The amount of this compound produced after 2 hour of treatment with base was approximately 0.50 mg (Table 3-5). No further hydroxytyrosol was produced after 24 hour consistent with its production from oleuropein and the complete destruction of oleuropein after 2 hour treatment with base. The amount of hydroxytyrosol produced by acid treatment (extraction and hydrolysis) increased significantly between 2 and 24 hour consistent with the extracts containing residual oleuropein at 2 hour. The amount of hydroxytyrosol that was produced after 24 hour acid-treatment was approximately 50 times that produced in basic extracts (Table 3-5).

3.2 Isolation and purification of oleuropein

3.2.1. Isolation and purification of oleuropein from olive leaves extract by column chromatography.

Column chromatography of the crude ethyl acetate extract of olive leaves allowed the isolation of the main phenolic compounds: oleuropein, hydroxytyrosol, verbascoside, luteolin 7-glucoside and oleuroside. The R_f values of the main compounds were determined to be 0.3-0.5 on a silica gel TLC plate using an organic layer of chloroform-methanol-water(13:7:4, v/v) mixture. Due to its polar nature, the methanol extract seemed ideally suited for further separation by liquid chromatography.

Structural determination by $[\alpha]_D$, UV, IR,[1][H] NMR showed that the major phenolic compound in ethyl acetate extract was oleuropein. This was confirmed by spectral studies on purified oleuropein obtained by this method which used in this study.

Oleuropein $[\alpha]_D^{28}$ = -146.2 °

UV: (EtOH) 228.5 nm (ξ = 18000), 278 nm (ξ = 3300).

IR (KBr): 3100-3500 (br OH), 1680-1725(br COO), 1620, 1520 (arom.) cm[1].

[1][H] NMR : 1.65 (3H,d) 2.41 (1H,dd), 2.63 (1H,dd), 2.69 (2H,t), 3.65 (3H,s,12–H), 3.86 (1H,dd,4-H), 3.95-4.18 (2H,m,8-H), 4.66 (1H,d,anomeric–H), 5.87 (1JH,s,2-H), 5.97 (1H,q,9-H), 6.48 (1H,dd,6-H), 6.66(1H,d,2-H), 6.65 (1H,d,5-H), 7.53 (1H,s,6-H), 8.73 (1H,d,OH).

3.2.2. Isolation and purification of oleuropein from olive leaves extract by RP-HPLC:

Five phenolic compounds were isolated using gradient solvent system (methanol/water) from 5.0 gm of ethyl acetate extract [(Luteolin 7- glucoside (25.0 mg) and verbascoside (825 mg), oleuropein (4000 mg) and oleuroside (133.6 mg) and rutin (16.4 mg)], and they were identified by comparison of their spectra with those of literature data [113]. The UV spectra of these extracts showed peaks at 280 and 330 nm that correspond to the absorption maxima of oleuropein and verbascoside, respectively as shown by figure (3-5).

The NMR instrument used in the identification of oleuropein is of Varian type.

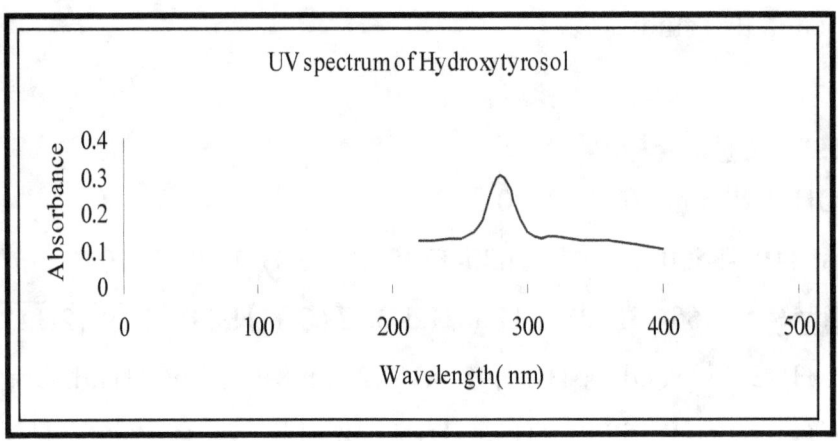

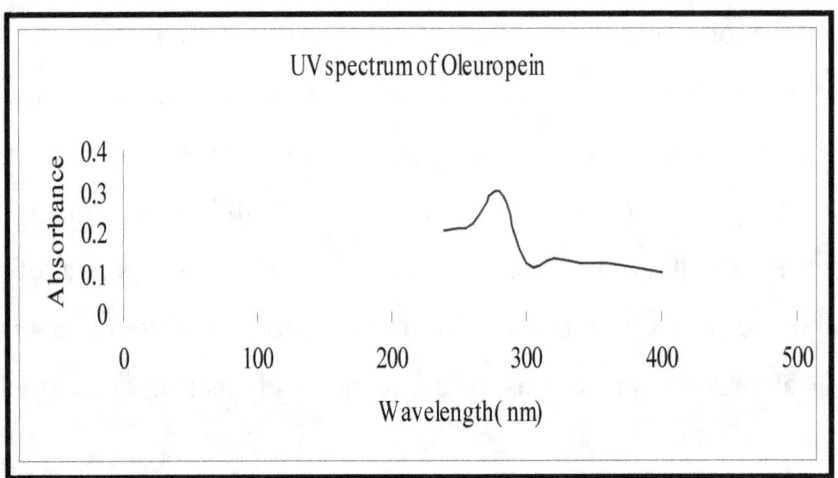

Figure 3-5. UV spectrum of major phenolic compounds isolated from Olive leaves extract.

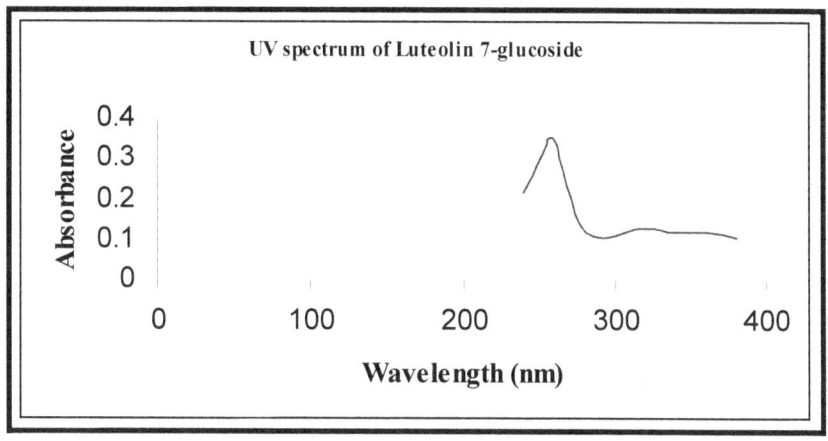

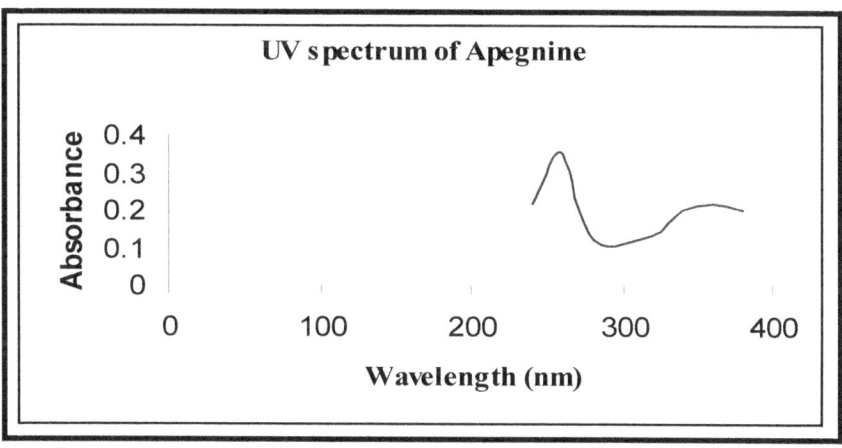

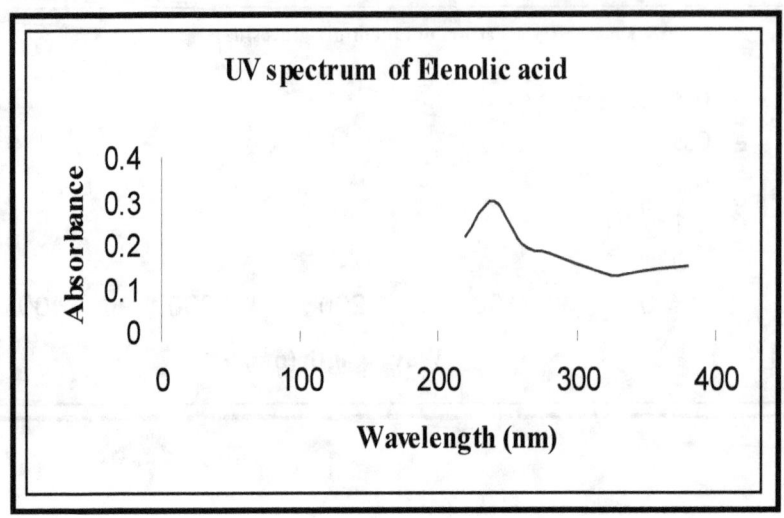

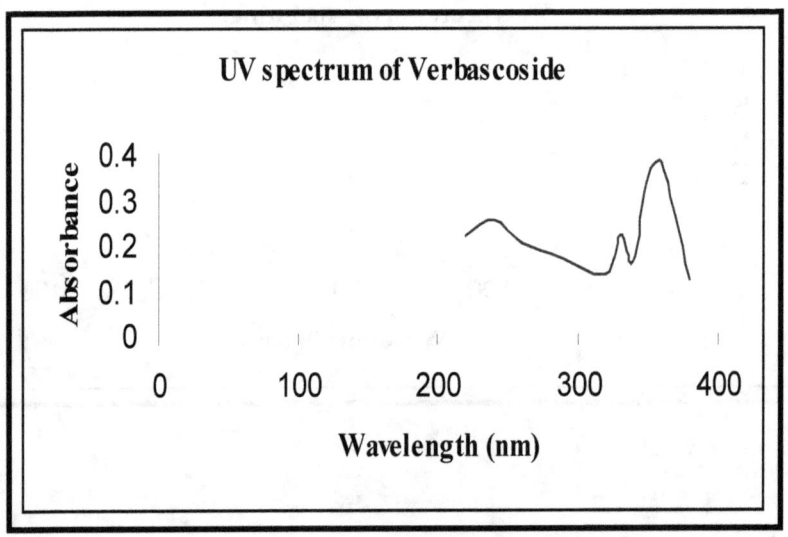

3.2.3. *Preparation of oleuropein aglycone from oleuropein*:

Oleuropein aglycone (OLEa) was prepared by enzymatic hydrolysis of oleuropein using β-glucosidase (from almonds) according to limiroli method [170]. The optimum conditions were pH = 7.4, incubation time =2 hour and incubation temperature = 60 °C. The oleuropein aglycone was isolated and purified as described by Limiroli et al (1995) using HPLC. The HPLC chromatogram of (OLEa) prepared was shown in the figure (3-6). Structural determination was confirmed by spectral studies UV, IR and [1] [H] NMR.

[1] **[H] NMR (CDCL$_3$)** : Significant protons at 9.60 and 9.50 (aldehyde protons); 6.80 and 6.55 (3H,m,s, phenyl protons), 3.70(3H, s, CH$_3$), 2.82(2H,t,C2-CH) ; 2.80(2H,t,CH$_2$),2.23(1 H,dd,C-CH$_2$), 1.51(3H,d,CH$_3$-CH).

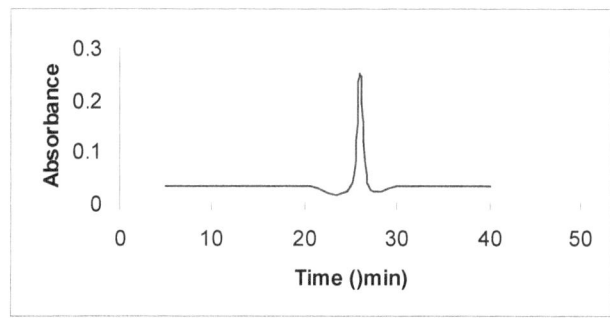

Figure   3-6. HPLC chromatogram of oleuropein aglycone.

The NMR analysis was carried out using Perkin –Elmer 60MHz, in College of science at Mosul University.

3.4. Preparation of elenolic acid from oleuropein aglycone.

Of particular interest because of its potent, broad range antiviral activity, the oleuropein related natural product elenolic acid which was assigned structure (in equilibrium with the open chain enol aldehyde and dialdehyde counterparts) by panizzi [2] was prepared by acid hydrolysis of oleuropein aglycone. The obtained crude elenolic acid was purified by column chromatography using silica gel 60 according to the method of Gardiobli [168]. Structural determination was confirmed by spectral studies UV, IR, and [1][H] NMR as shown in table 3-6.

Table 3-6.[1] [H] NMR spectrum of elenolic acid prepared by acid hydrolysis of oleuropein aglycone.

Line position (ppm)	Pattern	Assignment
1.58	Doublet	$CH_3 C(O) H$
4.28	Doublet of quartets	$CHC(O) HCH_3$
2.72	Multiplet	$C(O) HCH(CH)CHO$
3.40	Doublet of doublets	$CHCH_2CO_2$
2.95		$CHCH_2CO_2$
2.37		
3.75	Singlet	CO_2CH_3
7.70	Doublet	Conjugated $C=CHO$
9.70	Doublet	$CHCHO$
9.92	Broad	CO_2 exchangeable

The NMR analysis was carried out using Perkin –Elmer 60M.Hz, in College of Science at Mosul University.

3.5. Biological activity of Oleuropein

3.5.1. LDL oxidation and inhibition test

Figure (3-7) presents the inhibitory effects of four representative compounds oleuropein, hydroxytyrosol; luteolin 7-glucoside and vitamin E), representing each of the four examined classes (secoiridoid, polyphenols. flavonoids, and tocopherols, respectively), against *in vitro* LDL values tended to stabilize after using of sixth hour of incubation time periods . Remarkable antioxidant activity was observed for hydroxytyrosol the most potent compound studied, while the others exhibited less. Several concentrations of the tested compound (i.e., 5, 10, and 20 µM) were used (Table 3-7) considering that 20 µM oleuropein, resulting in approximately 50% mean protection (MP), is the usual reference. These concentrations indicated the limits of the protection activity of each compound. All of the examined compounds exhibited remarkable protection at 20µM final concentration with activity ranging from 34 % to 55.7 % (Table 3-8).

In table (3-7) the %MP values for oleuropein in concentration of 5, 10, 20 and 30 µM are presented. These values were obtained by applying the thiobarbituric acid reactant substances (TBARS) values to the ox- LDL test, where a dose dependent increment of % MP was observed. The 20 µM concentration of oleuropein has been reported as the dose above which the inhibitory effect is not significantly increased; it is therefore characterized as the highest optimal dose for this compound. Hydroxytyrosol and oleuropein and their derivatives which are the major polyphenols of olive leaf extract, olive oil, along with other polyphenols have been reported to have remarkable activity against LDL-oxidation either by copper ions or by other oxidizing agents[8]. The monitored LDL protective activity of oleuropein in present study was comparable to that reported previously by Visioli F et al (1994). Rutin and Luteolin are minor flavonoids polyphenol mainly found in olive leaf their relatively high LDL protection activity was found to be very close to oleuropein. These results obtained from our study for the flavonoids listed are comparable to those previously reported regarding the inhibitory effect against copper induced LDL oxidation. The biological activity of the minor flavonoids examined along with those previously reported could be considered to contribute to the beneficial effect of the major polyphenols against coronary heart disease enhancing the beneficial effect of the Mediterranean diet rich in olive oil.

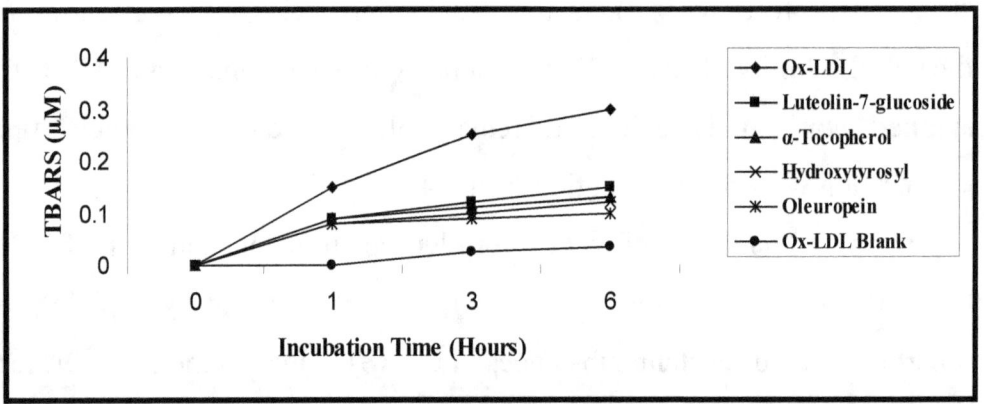

Figure 3-7. Biological activity of major olive leaf extract constituents (final concentration 20 μM) with various structure configurations expressed as ox-LDL inhibition.

Table 3-7. Inhibitory effect of oleuropein on LDLoxidation (ox-LDL) expressed as thiobarbituric acid reactant substances (TBARS M ± SD) and percent mean protection (%MP).

Test No.[a]	Test	1 hour	3 hour	6 hour	% MP[b]
-	Ox-LDL	1.412±0.08	2.293±0.26	2.694±0.26	0.0
1	OLE(5µM)	1.262±0.15	1.562±0.08	1.390±0.221	27.6
2	OLE(10µM)	1.191±0.11	1.295±0.09	1.213±0.11	35.8
3	OLE (20µM)	1.09±0.11	1.174±0.15	0.921±0.15	43.9
4	OLE (30µM)	1.189±0.12	1.294±0.09	1.210±0.12	36.0
-	oxLDL-Blank	0.0003	0.1000±0.08	0.223±0.08	95.4

[a]/ Tests 1, 2 ,3 and 4 consisted of the ox -LDL test with the addition of oleuropein in the concentration indicated. For ox-LDL and ox-LDL-blank tests, see Materials and Methods.

[b]/ The % MP is calculated from the values for Pt, the protection measured in each incubation period t ($t = 1$, 3, or 6), as follows. For each test number i; ($i= 1, 2,,3$ or 4), $Pt = (Nt - TBARSt)/Nt$, where $TBARSt$ = measured $TBARS$ value in µM) for test number i in incubation period t and the net oxidation Nt = (TBARS value of oxLDL test-TBARS value of oxLDL- blank test) in incubation period t. % MP is equal to the average Pt for all three tests expressed as a percentage: % MP = $\{\{\sum[Pt)i]\}/3\}*100$. For example, for oleuropein 20 µM test 3, N1 = (1.4121 -0.0003) = 1.4118, N3 = (2.2936-0.1) =2.1936, N6 = (2.6943-0.2233) = 2.4710; P1 = (1.4118 - 1.0917)/1.4118 = 0.2267, P3= (2.1936 - 1.1740)/2.1936 =0.4648, P6 = (2.4710 - 0.9212)/2.4710 =0.6271, and % MP = [(0.2267 ± 0.4648 ± 0.6271)/3]*100 = 43.9.

Table 3-8. Inhibitory effect of major olive leaf extract constituents on *in vitro* LDL oxidation expressed as percent Mean Protection (%MP).

Conc. (µM)	Rutin	Hydroxytyrosol	Luteolin 7-glucoside	Vit E(control)
5 µM	13.7	16.8	21.8	27.3
10 µM	40.2	55.7	38.6	35.8
20 µM	42.3	50.5	37.5	43.9
30 µM	43.3	46.6	23.6	33.7

3.5.2. Antioxidant test using APPH induced RBC hemolysis

Oleuropein, hydroxytyrosol, elenolic, rutin and luteolin 7-glucoside were tested for their effect on free radical induced hemolysis of RBC. Our results demonstrated that oleuropein, hydroxytyrosol and elenolic acid showed strong antioxidant effects (IC50 = 9.3 –37.5µM). Compound hydroxytyrosol exhibited the most potent activity (IC50 =9.3 µM), which was 4 times stronger than that Trolox. The activity of oleuropein and elenolic acid was also stronger than that of Trolox, but slightly weaker than that of hydroxytyrosol while, rutin and luteolin 7-glucoside showed weaker activity than Trolox. The IC50 of later compounds exceeded 200 μM. These experimental results suggested that the hemolysis inhibitory effect of these compounds might be related to the number of their phenolic hydroxyl groups (Figure 3-8).

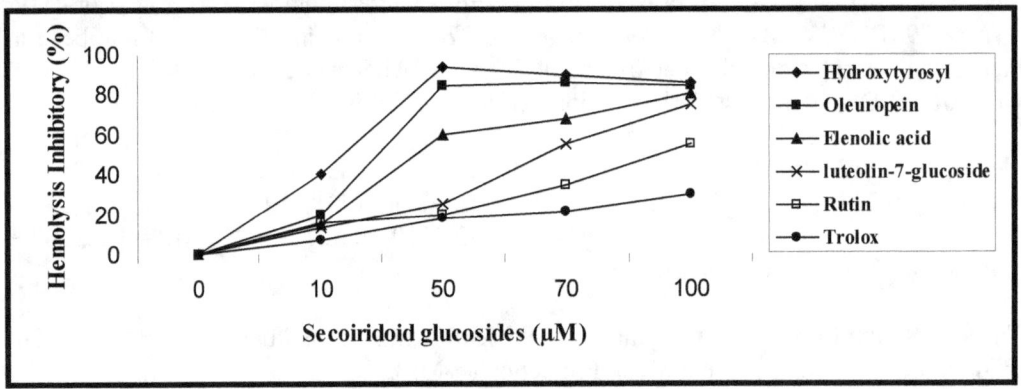

Figure 3-8. Inhibitory effect of individual Secoiridoids on APPH induced hemolysis of rabbit RBC in vitro.

3.5.3. Scavenging activity test of oleuropein using ABTS radical

The ABTS scavenging activity of olive leaf polyphenolic compound (oleuropein, hydroxytyrosol, oleuropein aglycone and vitamin E (as control) are reported in table (3-9). The total equivalent antioxidant capacity (TEAC) values showed that the olive leaf phenolic compounds were similar in their ability to scavenge the ABT radical cation. Reaction with ABTS/radical cation was complete after 1 min for all compounds tested.

Table3-9. Trolox equivalent antioxidant capacity (TEAC values) of phenolic compounds isolated from olive leaf extract determined by the 2,2-azobis(3-ethylbenzothiazoline-6-sulfonic acid) diammonium salt (ABTS) .

Compound	n	TEAC(*mmol/ L)*
Oleuropein	4	0.92 ± 0.02
Oleuropein aglycone	4	0.93 ± 0.02
Hydroxytyrosol	4	0.92 ± 0.02
Vit E.	4	0.90 ± 0.03

3.5.4. *Effect of oleuropein on glucose uptake in fat cells isolated from rabbit*

Insulin increases the rate of glucose transport across many cell membranes as illustrated in the figure (3-9) by measuring the rate of removal of glucose from the incubation medium by isolated fat cells, in this case membrane transport is the rate limiting step in glucose metabolism by the cells, so that an increase in the rate of removal of glucose from the medium is taken as indicating stimulation of glucose transport across the fat cell membrane. To know more details about the mechanism in which oleuropein reduce the levels of blood glucose in alloxan diabetic rabbits we designed the same experiment for insulin effect, and as shown in figure (3-10) there is a significant effect of oleuropein on glucose uptake, this action leads to conclude that oleuropein may be acts like insulin activity.

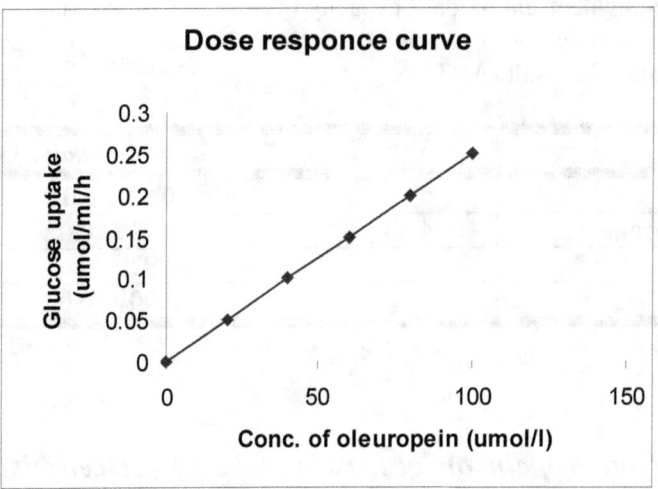

Figure 3-10. Effect of different concentrations of oleuropein on glucose uptake in fat cells Isolated from healthy rabbits.

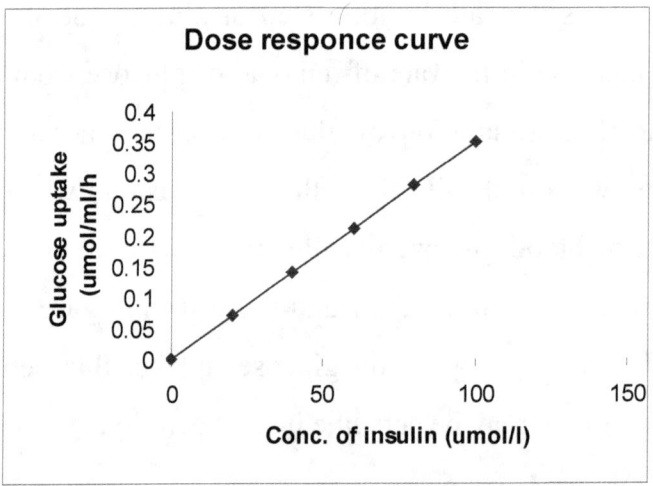

Figure 3-9. Dose response curve of insulin on glucose uptake isolated from healthy rabbits.

3.6. Animal Studies

3.6.1. Prophylactic effect of crude oleuropein in alloxan rabbits

The daily oral treatment with alloxan in a dose 150 mg/kg resulted in the development of diabetes after one week of administration, the effect gradually increasing over four week period to reach a rise of a bout two times % over initial values compared with normal rabbit. Rabbit administrated alloxan showed hyperglycemia ($p < 0.001$) at week 2 and 4), a significant $p < 0.05$ weight loss by week 2 and both polydipsia by the end of the study period 4 week (Table 3-10). Administration with 20 mg/kg daily crude oleuropein reduced the weight loss and polydipsia significantly ($p < 0.05$) at 4 weeks) associated with alloxan treatment. The concomitant use of the crude oleuropein of 20 mg/kg was not effective in suppressing the rise in blood sugar induced by alloxan, where in a dose of 50 mg/ kg , it was capable of reducing the rise in blood sugar induced by alloxan from (350 ± 9.9 mg/dl) to (200 ± 7.6 mg/dl) by the end of 4 weeks , it was evident, that the use of the 100 mg/kg dose of the leaf extract (crude oleuropein) had completely prevented the rise in blood sugar induced by alloxan (Table 3-10), as shown by the lack of statistical significance at $p < 0.05$ between that group and the normal control one.

Table 3-10. The effect of crude oleuropein (0, 20, 50, and 100 mg/kg) on body weight, fluid intake and blood sugar in alloxan induced diabetic and normal rabbits.

Parameter	Time (wk)	Control	Alloxan	20 mg/kg	50 mg/kg	100mg/kg)
Body Wt (g)	0	835 ± 27	810 ± 31	850±29	834 +33	823±31
	2	870 ±13	708 ± 21	821±21	821±24	800 ±24
	4	825 ± 32	700 ± 24	800 ±24	810 ±22	823 ±20
Fluid intake ml/day	0	40 ± 2.5	43 ± 2.4	41±7.2	40 ±2.6	43±1.5
	2	42 ± 1.8	58 ± 2.1	52±1.8	50 ±2.3	47 ±2.9
	4	43 ± 1.5	68 ± 4.6	43±1.5	45 ±4.4	44 ±4.3
B.sugar mg/dl	0	118 ± 9.5	116 ±7.8	117±8.1	119±9.2	117±8.1
	2	112 ± 7.8	250 ± 10	180±7.9	160 ± 6.6	140 ±7.1
	4	119 ± 8.2	350 ±9.9	260±10	200 ±7.6	120 ±7.7

3.6.2. Effects of each crude and pure oleuropein administration in alloxan rabbits.

The present study was carried out on alloxan induced diabetic rabbits to examine the effect of the daily intake of 20 mg crude or pure OLE on fasting blood sugar for a period of time (16 weeks). A significant decrease in blood sugar levels was observed in diabetic rabbits receiving daily 20 mg pure OLE through a different period of time per day, week, and month. A positive effect of OLE was very clear as shown in tables (3-11, 12, 13 and 14).

The pure OLE was more affected than crude OLE in lowering glucose levels in diabetic animals, so the interpretation of this difference may be attributed to less amount of OLE present in the crude extract and the action of the active constituent of olive leaf extract belonged to OLE, therefore in all further animal experiments a pure OLE had been used in order to study the positive effect of its biological activity in reducing hyperglycemia and lipid profile. Our results are in consistent with that reported by Gonzalez and others who found a hypoglycemic activity of aqueous olive leaf extract and they attributed this effect to oleuropein compound through two mechanisms (a): potentiation of glucose induced insulin release and (b) increased peripheral uptake of glucose [10, 26, and 27].

Table 3-11. Levels of fasting blood sugar (Mean ± SD in mg/dl) in alloxan diabetic rabbits receiving 20 mg of crude and pure oleuropein daily during 24 hr.

Time (h)	n	Normal rabbit		Alloxan diabetic rabbit	
		Crude OLE	*Pure OLE*	*Crude OLE*	*Pure OLE*
0	8	115 ± 4.2	113 ± 4.7	350 ± 7.3	347 ± 5.8
2	8	94 ± 4.3	90 ± 3.9	320 ± 6.7	280 ± 7.2
4	8	88 ± 5.3	80 ± 4.1	300 ± 5.7	233 ± 6.6
6	8	90 ± 4.4	86 ± 3.9	310 ± 4.9	250 ± 5.8
12	8	99 ± 5.2	100 ± 3.7	320 ± 5.2	261 ± 4.7
24	8	105 ± 4.2	102 ± 3.6	324 ± 4.8	270 ± 5.2

Table 3-12. Levels of fasting blood sugar (Mean ± SD in mg/dl) in alloxan diabetic rabbits receiving 20 mg of crude and pure OLE daily during one week.

DAY	n	Alloxan rabbits treated with crude oleuropein	Alloxan rabbits treated with pure oleuropein
1	8	325 ± 7.6	270 ± 5.2
2	8	310 ± 5.8	261 ± 6.2
3	8	290 ± 6.7	254 ± 5.6
4	8	280 ± 7.5	248 ± 6.3
5	8	271 ± 4.9	232 ± 7.1
6	8	259 ± 5.3	217 ± 6.2
7	8	245 ± 6.7	212 ± 5.6

Table 3-13. Levels of fasting blood sugar (Mean ± SD in mg/dl) in alloxan diabetic rabbits receiving 20 mg of crude and pure OLE daily during 5 weeks.

Week	n	Alloxan rabbits treated with crude oleuropein	Alloxan rabbits treated with pure oleuropein
1	8	245 ± 6.7	212 ± 5.6
2	8	234 ± 4.7	202 ± 4.3
3	8	230 ± 4.2	190 ± 3.9
4	8	211 ± 4.1	181 ± 3.8
5	8	200 ± 3.9	171 ± 3.3

Table 3-14. Levels of fasting blood sugar (Mean ± SD in mg/dl) in alloxan diabetic rabbits receiving 20 mg daily of crude and pure OLE during 4 months.

Month	n	Alloxan treated with crude oleuropein	Alloxan treated with pure oleuropein
1	8	200 ± 3.9	171 ± 3.3
2	8	181 ± 4.2	160 ± 6.7
3	8	170 ± 3.9	142 ± 4.1
4	8	161 ± 3.6	133 ± 3.9

3.6.3. Effect of OLE intake on blood glucose levels in alloxan induced diabetic rabbits and human NIDDM patients.

As shown in table 3-15 a significant decrease in the levels of blood sugar (133 ± 3.9) mg /dl were obtained in alloxan induced diabetic rabbits receiving 20 mg of pure OLE daily for 16 week compared with (350 ± 11.8) mg/ dl before treatment. These results are compatible with experiment done with NIDDM patients as shown in table 3-16 .The levels of blood sugar in NIDDM patients administrated 1.0 gm OLE daily for 6 months are decreased significantly $p<0.001$ (155 ± 8.8) mg/dl compared with (250 ± 9.6)) mg/dl in those patients before OLE intake. The persistence of hyperglycemia in NIDDM patients under study leads to an increase of oxidative stress by several mechanism including glucose autooxidation and non-enzymatic protein glycation, as well as the same condition occurred in alloxan induced diabetic rabbits, so the positive effect of OLE may be investigate more details of more than one mechanism.

OLE act by decreasing insulin resistance at the level of muscle and fat, so that the body owns insulin becomes more efficient in its action to control blood glucose. OLE do not cause low blood glucose (hypoglycemia) but in combination with other agent such as glipizide. The peak blood glucose lowering effect is seen at 4hr underlying the insulin releasing action of OLE argue against an action similar to sulphonylurea drugs, currently used for diabetic therapy. These agents may be act by binding to sulphonylurea receptors resulting in closure of the membrane K-ATP channels, depolarization of membrane opening of voltage-dependent calcium channels and elevation of intracellular calcium ions. Possible actions of OLE may include enhancement of β-cell glucose metabolism or activation of enzyme systems generating cyclic AMP or phospholipids derived messengers in conclusion, the antihyperglycemic action of OLE is associated with the stimulation of insulin secretion and improvement sensitivity of insulin.

Our data agree well with that reported by some researchers who found that the natural olive leaf compounds can decrease the levels of blood sugar Our data agree also well with that reported by Onderoglu [26] who observed that significant decreases in some biochemical and hematological parameters of streptozotocin treated rats such as, glucose, GPT, urea, cholesterol, GOT, no visible toxicity except/decrease in body weight gain attributable to long term use of plant materials. These data indicate that long term use of olive leaf may provide benefit effects against diabetic conditions. From clinical report by Privitera 1998, one involved a 15-year-old girl with juvenile diabetes. The teenager had been regularly taking 35 units of insulin daily for control. After one month on olive leaf extract, she was able to maintain similar control with just 12 units. In another case, the blood sugar level of a diabetic elderly patient dropped from 450 to 160 mg/dl after three months. In a yet another instance, the blood sugar of a middle aged man stabilized at 140, down from 250, after one month [1].

Table 3–15. Levels of blood sugar (Mean ± SD) in healthy and alloxan diabetic rabbits after long term administration of 20 mg OLE daily for 16 weeks.

Group	n	Blood sugar (mg/dl)	T- test
Healthy Rabbits	8	120 ± 11.2	
Alloxan diabetic rabbits pre-OLE intake	8	350 ± 12.7	P <0.001
Alloxan diabetic rabbits post-OLE take	8	133 ± 3.9	P <0.001

Table 3-16. Levels of blood sugar (Mean ±SD) in healthy and NIDDM patients after long term administration of 1.0 gm OLE daily for 6 months.

Group	n	Blood sugar (mg/dl)	T-test
Healthy subjects	25	110 ± 8.9	
NIDDM patients pre-OLE intake	30	250 ± 9.6	P< 0.001
NIDDM patients post-OLE intake	30	155 ± 8.8	P< 0.001

3.6.4. Effect of OLE intake on serum total cholesterol levels in alloxan induced diabetic rabbits and NIDDM patients.

The levels of serum total cholesterol was significantly reduced p< 0.001 (60 ± 3.8) mg/dl in alloxan diabetic rabbits receiving 20 mg of pure OLE daily for 16 week compared with the levels (90 ± 4.5) mg/dl in diabetic rabbits without treatment as shown in table 3-17.

From table 3-18 we noticed that there is significant increase in the levels of total cholesterol in NIDDM patients p< 0.001 (300 ± 9.7) mg/ dl compared with (221 ± 8.7) mg/dl in healthy subjects. Our data are consistent with that reported by researchers who attributed this increase of total cholesterol levels to oxidative stress conditions which had been occurred in NIDDM and positively correlated with a long period of the disease, in addition to a defect in LDL receptor as a result of glycation of a receptor. When the NIDDM patients intake 1.0 gm of OLE for a long time (6 months) the levels of total cholesterol were decreased from (300 ± 9.7) mg/dl to (240 ± 6.6) mg/dl after treatment . OLE showed a hypolipidmic agent in reducing total cholesterol and other lipid profile. Our data conducted with that reported by Coni who found that when diabetic rabbits intake olive oil plus OLE in their diet a significant decrease in total cholesterol was obtained [12].

Table 3-17. Levels of total cholesterol (Mean ± SD) in healthy and alloxan diabetic rabbits after long term administration of 20 mg OLE daily for 16 weeks.

Group	n	T. cholesterol (mg/dl)	T- test
Healthy rabbits	8	40 ± 3.2	
Alloxan diabetic rabbits pre-OLE intake	8	90 ±4.5	P <0.001
Alloxan diabetic rabbits post-OLE intake	8	60 ±3.8	P <0.001

Table 3-18. Levels of total cholesterol (Mean ± SD) in healthy subjects and NIDDM patients after long term administration of 1.0 gm OLE daily for 6 months.

Group	n	T-cholesterol (mg/dl)	T- test
Healthy Subjects	25	221 ± 11.2	
NIDDM patients pre-OLE intake	30	300 ± 9.7	P <0.001
NIDDM patients post-OLE intake	30	240 ± 11.2	P <0.001

3.6.5. Effect of oleuropein intake on serum HDL-c levels in alloxan induced diabetic and NIDDM patients

Table 3-19 showed a significant decrease in the levels of HDL-c $p < 0.001$ (7.5± 1.1) mg/dl in alloxan diabetic rabbits after 16 week of onset the disease,, compared with (13 ± 2.1) mg/dl in control non diabetic rabbit , while these levels of cholesterol increased to normal baseline levels (11 ± 1.7) mg/dl when alloxan diabetic rabbits receiving 20 mg of pure OLE daily a long that time period, these results observed a positive effect of OLE intake with a long period of time used. On the other hand significant decrease of HDL-c in NIDDM patients $p<0.001$(32 ± 3.6) mg/dl compared with (55± 4.7) mg/dl in healthy subjects, while these levels were increased to (45 ± 4.2) mg/dl in NIDDM patients after intake 1.0 gm of OLE daily for 6 months, as it was shown in table (3-20).

This decrease associated with duration diabetic period in NIDDM which may increase atherosclerosis conditions due to the importance of HDL in transfer cholesterol from cells to the liver, the mechanism of this decrease in HDL in NIDDM patients may be explained by increase levels of MDA, and an increase in the activity of ETP enzyme which transfer cholesterol ester from HDL to VLDL and leave HDL rich in triglyceride easily filtered by kidney. These results agree well with that reported by Ginberg [219]. Other studies explain the mechanism of decreasing levels in NIDDM patients by alteration in liver function which inhibit production of apo-Al protein as well as presence of high levels of MDA due to lipid peroxidation process and low levels of polyunsaturated fatty acids leads to increase in the activity of ETP [220].

Other studies observed that there is an inverse relationship between activity of CETP and the levels of HDL which leads to reduce atherosclerosis [217,221]. Reducing levels of apo-protein (A) leads to reduce the LACT activity secreted by liver which act on transfer of fatty acid from lecithin to free cholesterol producing ester cholesterol resulting in reducing HDL in blood [223,224]. Administration of 1.0 gm oleuropein daily for 6 months by NIDDM patients improved levels of HDL-c from (32 ± 3.6) mg/dl before treatment to (45 ± 4.2) mg/dl after OLE intake. This improvement may be due to improved glycemic control and inhibition of lipid peroxidation process, low levels of MDA and balance of oxidant/antioxidant condition due to antioxidant and biological activity of oleuropein, and its metabolite hydroxyl tyrosol, so OLE is considered a protective compound for cardiovascular disease, which was one danger complication of diabetic disease. These results agree well with that reported that olive oil supplementation reduced the incidence of CHD [11].

The effects of OLE intake on plasma lipids agree with that reported by Bonanome [225] that diets rich in olive oil raise the resistance of plasma LDL to oxidative modification as well as Visioli [226] who found that natural antioxidant (polyphenolic compounds) of olive oil inhibited the formation cytotoxic products such as LDL- lipid peroxides, thus retarding the onset of atherosclerosis damage.

Table 3-19. Levels of HDL-c (Mean $\pm$ SD) in healthy and alloxan induced diabetic rabbits after long term administration of 20 mg OLE daily for 16 weeks.

Group	n	HDL-c (mg/dl)	T- test
Healthy rabbits	8	7.5 ± 1.1	
Alloxan diabetic rabbits pre-OLE intake	8	13 ± 2.1	P< 0.001
Alloxan diabetic rabbits post-OLE intake	8	11 ± 1.7	P< 0.001

Table 3-20. Levels of HDL-c (Mean ± SD) in healthy subjects and NIDDM after long term administration of 1.0 gm OLE daily for 6 months.

Group	n	HDL-c (mg/dl)	T- test
Healthy subjects	25	55 ± 4.7	
NIDDM patients pre-OLE intake	30	32 ± 3.6	P < 0.001
NIDDM patients post-OLE intake	30	45 ± 4.2	P < 0.001

3.6.6. Effect of OLE intake on serum LDL-c levels in alloxan induced diabetic rabbits and NIDDM patients

A significant increase was obtained in alloxan diabetic rabbits after 16 week of onset the disease P < 0.001 (76 ± 4.4) mg/dl compared with (24 ± 3.3) mg/dl in non diabetic rabbits. These levels of cholesterol were decreased from (76 ± 4.4) mg./dl to (45 ± 3.3) mg/dl after intake 20 mg OLE daily for 16 week, as shown in table (3-21). A significant increase in levels of cholesterol LDL was seen in NIDDM patients p <0.001 (165 ± 10.5) mg/dl compared with (90 ± 9.5)mg/dl healthy subjects , while it was reduced to(120 ± 9.4) mg/dl after long term administration of 1.0 gm OLE daily for 6 months as shown in table (3- 22).

This increase in LDL levels in NIDDM patients was due to an increased lipid per-oxidation process which stimulated by hyperglycemia and a consequence of these events defect in LDL-receptors taken place. Our results agree well with that reported by Visioli [226] .Oxidation of low density lipoprotein (LDL) cholesterol is a key step in the formation of atheroma and is thought to be a major factor in the development of cardiovascular disease. This may be of particular importance in patients with NIDDM, in addition to raised total LDL cholesterol levels; they tend to have a pro-atherogenic lipid profile composed of small dense LDL particles, raised triglycerides and moderately raised cholesterol. Small dense LDL particles are known to be more readily oxidized than larger particles, partly because they have less protective vitamin E. Once modified, they are taken up by macrophages in the arterial intimae via the scavenger receptor, eventually forming foam cells, which predispose to the formation of atherosclerotic plaques [11].

Consumption of OLE inhibited the progression of atherosclerosis; this effect was associated with a significant reduction in the plasma and LDL cholesterol levels. Atherosclerosis is a multifactorial disease associated with different risk factors, hypercholesterolemia is a major risk factor for atherosclerosis and reduction in plasma cholesterol levels by drug therapy has reduced cardiovascular incidence. Consumption of natural nutrients capable of reducing plasma cholesterol, thus showed also reduces development of atherosclerosis [227].

Our study demonstrated that dietary consumption of OLE by alloxan, diabetic rabbits significantly reduced development of aortic atherosclerosis, along with an impressive reduction in the levels of plasma and LDL cholesterol. The hypolipidmic and anti atherosclerosis effects of OLE could have possibly resulted at least in part, from the inhibition of cellular cholesterol biosynthesis observed after consumption of OLE, suggesting that in vivo following consumption and digestion, cellular cholesterol synthesis may be inhibited by some OLE derived metabolite. Reduced cellular cholesterol biosynthesis is associated with increased activity of the LDL-receptor resulting in enhanced removal of LDL from plasma resulting in reduced plasma cholesterol concentration. These results are in agreement with previously reported data showing that plant food possesses cholesterol suppressive capacity. We conclude that consumption of OLE may be proven beneficial in attenuation of atherosclerosis development since it reduced oxidative state of LDL and reduced LDL per-oxidation; all these effects lead to a reduced cellular cholesterol accumulation and foam cell formation the hallmark of early atherosclerosis. The effects of OLE intake on plasma lipids agree with that reported by Bonanome [225] reported that diets rich in olive oil raise the resistance of plasma LDL to oxidative modification. Visioli et al 1995 found that natural antioxidant (polyphenolic compounds) contained in olive oil inhibited the formation of cytotoxic products such as LDL lipid peroxides, thus retarding the onset of atherosclerosis damage [226].

Table 3-21. Levels of LDL-c (Mean ±SD) in healthy and alloxan diabetic rabbits after long administration of 20 mg OLE daily for 16 weeks.

Group	n	LDL-c (mg/dl)	T- test
Healthy rabbits	8	24 ± 3.2	
Alloxan diabetic rabbits pre-OLE intake	8	76 ± 4.4	P< 0.001
Alloxan diabetic rabbits post-OLE intake	8	45 ± 3.3	P< 0.001

Table 3-22. Levels of LDL-c (Mean ±SD) in healthy subjects and NIDDM after daily administration of 1.0 gm OLE for 6 months.

Group	n	LDL-c (mg/dl)	T- test
Healthy subjects	25	90 ± 8.5	
NIDDM patients pre- OLE intake	30	165 ± 10.5	P< 0.001
NIDDM patients post-OLE intake	30	120 ± 9.4	P< 0.001

3.6.7. Effect of OLE intake on serum VLDL-c levels in alloxan induced diabetic rabbits and NIDDM patients.

Table (3-23) shows that levels of VLDL-c significantly increased in alloxan diabetic rabbits p< 0.05 (6.1 ± 0.18) mg/dl compared with (3.2 ± 0.22) mg/ dl in healthy rabbits, while these levels decreased 30% when the alloxan diabetic rabbits receiving 20 mg of OLE daily for 16 week. Similar data had been obtained in NIDDM patients. Levels of VLDL were increased significantly $p < 0.001$ (36 ± 3.5) mg/dl compared with (27 ± 3.1) mg/ dl in healthy subjects (Table 3-24).

This increase in levels of VLDL in NIDDM patients is due to poor metabolic control and lipid profile re-distribution taken place in diabetes disease. Other causes of increase associated with causes leads to elevated triglyceride levels. The intake OLE by NIDDM patients for 6 months period reduced VLDL levels from (36 ± 3.5) mg/dl to (29 ± 2.8) mg/dl due to decreased levels of triglycerides. Our results are in agreement with that reported by Coni and Carmen [12,228].

Table 3-23. Levels of VLDL-c (Mean ± SD) in healthy and alloxan diabetic rabbits after long term administration of 20 mg OLE daily for l6 weeks.

Group	n	VLDL-c(mg/dl)	T- test
Healthy rabbits.	8	3.2 ± 0.22	
Alloxan diabetic rabbits pre-OLE intake	8	6.1 ± 0.44	P< 0.05
Alloxan diabetic rabbits post-OLE intake	8	4.2 ± 0.18	P< 0.05

Table 3-24. Levels of VLDL-c (Mean ± SD) in healthy subjects and NIDDM after long term administration of 1.0 gm OLE daily for 6 months.

Group	n	VLDL-c(mg/dl)	T- test
Healthy subjects	25	27 ± 3.1	
NIDDM patients pre- OLE intake	30	36 ± 3.6	P< 0.05
NIDDM patients post- OLE intake	30	29 ± 2.8	P< 0.05

3.6.8. *Effect of OLE intake on serum triglycerides levels in alloxan induced diabetic rabbits and NIDDM patients*

Table (3-25) showed a significant increase in levels of serum triglycerides in alloxan diabetic rabbits $p<0.001$ (30 ± 3.3) mg/dl compared with (15 ± 2.1) mg/dl in nondiabetic rabbits, while these levels decreased from (30 ± 3.3), mg/dl to (20 ± 2.5) mg/dl after receiving 20 mg of OLE daily for 16 week. The same results were obtained in human NIDDM patients (Table 3-26). Triglyceride levels in NIDDM patients were increased significantly p <0.001 (210 ± 13.5) mg/dl compared with (110 ± 12.5) mg/dl in healthy subjects. This increase may be due to a variety of metabolic abnormalities such as lipolysis process which happened in order to liberates of ATP as a source of energy although a hyperglycemia condition present. A deficiency of insulin levels in diabetic disease leads to increase lipid per-oxidation which effect on the activity of (LPL enzyme, this decrease in LPL activity leads to increase of triglyceride levels in NIDDM [224]. After administration of OLE for a long time by NIDDM patients improved oxidative stress condition and less free radical liberated, less MDA liberated. [228]

Table 3-25. Levels of serum triglycerides (Mean ± SD) in healthy and alloxan diabetic rabbits after long administration of 20 mg OLE daily for 16 weeks.

Group	n	Serum TG (mg/dl)	T- test
Healthy rabbits	8	15 ± 2.1	
Alloxan diabetic rabbits pre-OLE intake	8	30 ± 3.3	P <0.001
Alloxan diabetic rabbits post- OLE intake	8	20 ± 2.5	P <0.001

Table 3-26. Levels of serum triglycerides (Mean ± SD) of healthy subjects and NIDDM after long administration of 1.0 gm OLE daily for 6 months.

Group	n	Serum TG (mg/dl)	T- test
Healthy subjects	25	110 ± 12.5	
NIDDM patients pre- OLE intake	30	210 ±13.3	P <0.001
NIDDM patients post- OLE intake	30	160 ±11.2	P <0.001

3.6.9. Effect of OLE intake on serum uric acid in alloxan induced diabetic rabbits and NIDDM patients.

Serum uric acid levels were increased significantly in alloxan diabetic rabbits $p<0.05$ (2.8 ± 0.31) mg/dl compared with healthy rabbits (1.8 ± 0.22) mg./dl, while these levels decreased in alloxan diabetic rabbits receiving 20 mg daily of OLE for 16 week to levels not significant from control group (2.0 ± 0.18) mg/dl as shown in table (3-27).

Serum uric acid levels were increased significantly $p<0.05$ in NIDDM patients (7.9 ± 0.33) mg/dl compared with healthy subjects (6.2 ± 0.61) mg/dl while in NIDDM patients receiving 1.0 gm daily of OLE for 6 months decreased to levels not significant from control group (6.5 ± 0.22) mg/dl as shown in table(3-28).

The results in this study agree well with that reported by Habeeb et al [229].The mechanism via hyperuricemia is associated with diabetes mellitus disease remain unexplained. Hyperuricemia could be an "innocent bystander," a nonspecific marker of adverse pattern of risk factors. However, we do not exclude the possibility that hyperuricemia could play a role the pathogenesis of atherosclerosis. Overwhelming evidence suggests that hyperuricemia is linked to obesity, [230] hypertension,[231]reduced HDL, hypertriglyceridemia [232] hyperinsulinemia and reduced insulin sensitivity components the metabolic syndrome[230,231]. We also observed this association and the presence of multiple risk factors is likely to explain a substantial part of increased risk of stroke. However, even after extensive adjustment for cardiovascular risk factors, serum uric acid remained an independent risk factor for stroke elevated levels of serum uric acid are due to either an increase in uric acid production or a decrease in its excretion. Differences in dietary purine intake are unlikely to explain the association of hyperuricemia with diabetes However, there are other physiological and pathological factors that influence serum uric acid levels. Ferris [233] demonstrated in normal subjects that sympathetic nervous system stimulation induced by nore-pinephrine or angiotensin II infusion caused a multianeous increase in serum uric acid levels and blood pressure. These changes were reversible after the discontinuation of the pressure agent, serum uric acid levels have been reported to be inversely related to renal blood flow and directly to renal vascular resistance in both normotensive and hypertensive humans.

Some researchers demonstrated that high uric acid levels were independently associated with increased proximal tubular sodium reabsorption in men [234-236]. This association is strikingly similar to the ability of insulin to promote renal sodium reabsorption that has been suggested to be one of the reasons for the high frequency of hypertension in metabolic syndrome and NIDDM [237].

In insulin-resistant states the vasodilatory effect insulin mediated by nitric oxide is blunted, leading to disturbances in arterial blood flow [237] .On the other hand, hyperuricemia has been associated with elevated circulating endothelin levels [238] and one of the major sites of the production of uric acid in the cardiovascular system is the vessel wall and particularly the endothelium [239]. Recently, Steinberg has demonstrated that cardiac autonomic neuropathy is an independent predictor of stroke in patients with NIDDM [238].

Toyry JP *et al* (1996) taken together, these findings suggest that high uric acid could also be a marker sodium retention coupled with impaired hemodynamic reserves and/or disturbed blood flow [240]. Uric acid is one of the major endogenous water-soluble antioxidants of the body. There is accumulating evidence that increased oxidative stress is closely related to diabetes and its vascular complications [241] thus, high circulating uric acid levels may be an indicator that the body is trying to protect itself from the deleterious effects of free radicals by increasing the products of endogenous antioxidants, e.g., uric acid. Interestingly, uric cid prevents oxidative modification of endothelial enzymes and preserves the ability of endothelium to mediate vascular dilatation in the face of oxidative stress [242].

There is also some evidence that uric acid may have a direct role in the atherosclerotic process, because human atherosclerotic plaque contains more uric acid than do control arteries [243-244]. Inflammation is one of the features of atherosclerosis and uric acid crystals may induce inflammatory responses that are reduced by lipoproteins which have an ability to bind uric acid crystals [245,246]. Hyperuricemia via purine metabolism may also promote thrombus formation [247,248]. Serum uric acid was measured only once, and we therefore have no information on the stability of uric acid levels over time. However, a single measurement of a parameter usually weakens the associations observed. In conclusion, our results suggest that hyperuricemia is a strong predictor of stroke events in middle-aged patients with NIDDM, and this association is independent of other cardiovascular risk factors. The mechanisms through which hyperuricemia increases the risk of stroke should be the focus so OLE intake had been shown a highly benefit in reducing levels of uric acid in NIDDM through increased blood flow and increased the total antioxidant capacity and alternatively less oxidative stress syndrome which is associated with DM disease.

Table 3-27. Levels of serum uric acid (Mean ± SD) in healthy and alloxan diabetic rabbits after long administration of 20 mg OLE daily for 16 weeks.

Group	n	Uric acid (mg/dl)	T- test
Healthy Rabbits	8	1.8 ± 0.22	
Alloxan diabetic rabbits pre-OLE intake	8	2.8 ± 0.31	P< 0.05
Alloxan diabetic rabbits post-OLE intake	8	2.0 ± 0.18	P< 0.05

Table 3-28. Levels of serum uric acid (Mean ± SD) in healthy subjects and NIDDM after long administration of 1.0 gm OLE daily for 6 months.

Group	n	Uric acid (mg/dl)	T- test
Healthy subjects	25	6.2 ± 0.61	
NIDDM patients pre- OLE intake	30	7.9 ± 0.33	P< 0.05
NIDDM patients post- OLE intake	30	6.5 ± 0.22	P< 0.05

3.6.10. Effect of OLE intake on glycated Hb in alloxan induced diabetic rabbits and NIDDM patients

From table 3-29 no significant change in levels of glycated hemoglobin in alloxan induced diabetic rabbits after 16 week from onset of diabetes compared with healthy rabbit in addition to similar results were obtained in alloxan diabetic rabbit receiving 20 mg of OLE daily for 16 week period. These data may be due to short time of diabetes disease in alloxan rabbits can not effected the levels of glycated hemoglobin although a hyperglycemia condition present and oxidative stress taken place, generation of free radicals and MDA increased as well as induction effect of antioxidant enzymes occurred in the first period of onset the disease. The levels of glycated hemoglobin is increased significantly in NIDDM patients p<0.001 (8.8 ± 1.2) % compared with healthy subjects. (4.5 ± 0.5)%., as a result of hyperglycemia condition present in NIDDM (Table 3-30).

Diabetic patients are exposed to increased oxidative stress due to several mechanisms including glucose auto-oxidation and non-enzymatic protein glycation. Non-enzymatic glycation is a spontaneous chemical reaction between glucose and the amino groups of proteins in which reversible shiff bases and more stable amadori products are formed [266]. Intracellular hyperglycemia may lead, via processes of glucose auto-oxidation to increase the generation of oxygen free radicals and glycation of some antioxidant enzymatic proteins [250].

Our studies have shown that OLE administration to NIDDM patients resulted in improvement the levels of glucose and lipid profile and antioxidant enzyme activities, so the levels of glycated hemoglobin is reduced from (8.8 ± 2.3) to (6.6 ± 1.2) in NIDDM patients after OLE intake for 6 month period, therefore determination of levels of glycated hemoglobin is considered a good indicator to investigate the effect of administration of OLE on NIDDM patients.

Table 3-29. Levels of HbA_{1C} (Mean ± SD) in healthy and alloxan diabetic rabbits after long term administration of 20 mg OLE daily for 16 weeks.

Group	n	HbA_{1C} (%)	T- test
Healthy rabbits	8	3.1 ± 0.23	
Alloxan diabetic rabbits pre-OLE intake	8	3.63 ± 0.18	N.S
Alloxan diabetic rabbits post OLE intake	8	3.32 ± 0.21	N.S

Table 3-30. Levels of HbA_{1C} (Mean ± SD) in healthy subjects and NIDDM patients after long term administration of 1.0 gm OLE daily for 6 months.

Group	n	HbA_{1C} (%)	T- test
Healthy subjects	25	4.5 ± 1.2	
NIDDM patients pre- OLE intake	30	8.8 ± 2.3	P <0.05
NIDDM patients post- OLE intake	30	6.6 ± 1.4	P <0.05

3.6.11. Effect of OLE intake on plasma and erythrocytes MDA levels in alloxan induced diabetic rabbits and NIDDM patients.

Erythrocyte MDA levels were increased significantly in alloxan diabetic rabbits p <0.001 to (3.99 ± 0.45) µmol/g Hb compared with (1.77 ± 0.35) µmol/g Hb in control non diabetic rabbits, in addition to these levels of MDA decreased to a similar base line of normal values in alloxan diabetic rabbit receiving 20 mg of OLE daily for 16 week period as shown in table (3-31).

On the other hand, erythrocyte MDA levels had been already increased significantly in NIDDM patients p <0.001 to (4.44 ± 0.65) µmol/ g Hb compared with that in control groups (2.22 ± 0.21), while the levels of erythrocyte MDA was significantly reduced in NIDDM patients to (2.66 ± 0.33) when 1.0 gm of OLE was administrated for 6 months compared with NIDDM patient at baseline before supplementation with OLE (Table 3-32).

This study demonstrated the elevated concentration of plasma MDA , an end product of polyunsaturated fatty acid per-oxidation 20 days after clinical onset of diabetes induced in rabbits by alloxan p <0.001 (11.5 ± 1.9) nmol/ml compared with (4.4 ± 0.66) nmol/ml in healthy rabbits. This suggests that oxygen free radicals may already have exerted their cytotoxic effects in this early clinical stage of the disease but intake of 20 mg of OLE for 16 week period by alloxan diabetic rabbit improved the oxidative stress and inhibited lipid per-oxidation process so low levels of MDA were present as shown in table (3-33).

The same view was obtained in measuring the levels of plasma MDA in NIDDM patients who had more than 10 year period of onset of diabetes. The levels marked increase (28.5 ± 5.5) nmol/ml compared with(3.6 ± 0.75) nmol/ml in healthy subjects, while these levels decreased from (28.5 ± 5.5) nmol/ml before treatment with OLE to (10.6 ± 3.6) nmol/ml after treatment with 1.0 gm of OLE daily for 6 month , as shown in table (3-34).

A significant increase in MDA content of erythrocytes of patients with NIDDM was found compared with the reference group which suggested permanent structural membrane alterations in diabetes and also increased production of reactive oxygen species in the circulation. We observed that further intensification of lipid per-oxidation taken place in NIDDM patients, this fact may indicate increased production of free radicals or diminished efficiency of antioxidant defense mechanism in diabetes compared with healthy subjects [251]

Several studies have reported significant increase in lipid peroxides by TBAR measurement in both type 1&2 diabetic patients [251-253], however spectrophotometric analysis of TBARs over estimate MDA content, since dialdehydes other than MDA and other plasma component reacts with TBA to form colored complexes, in fact the limited specificity of this method is the main reason for questioning the validity of TBARS in evaluating the presence of oxidative stress. In NIDDM patients receiving 1.0 gm of OLE the MDA levels decreased from (4.44 ± 0.65) μmol/g Hb to a (2.66 ± 0.33) μmol/g Hb after 6 month of treatment due to the positive effect of OLE in inhibition of lipid per-oxidation, so low levels of MDA are present. Improvement of total antioxidant capacity, glycemic control and oxidative stress in NIDDM is a positive benefit of this polyphenolic compound in olive leaf. Our data agree well with that reported by Visioli et al (1998), who found that OLE inhibited lipid per-oxidation of LDL [11].

Table 3-31. Levels of Malondialdehyde (Mean ± SD) in erythrocytes of healthy and alloxan diabetic rabbits patients after long term administration of 20 mg OLE daily for 16 weeks.

Group	n	MDA (μmol/g Hb)	T- test
Healthy rabbits	8	1.77 ± 0.33	
Alloxan diabetic rabbits pre-OLE intake	8	3.99 ± 0.43	P< 0.001
Alloxan diabetic rabbits post OLE intake	8	1.93 ± 0.35	P< 0.001

Table 3-32. Levels of Malondialdehyde (Mean ± SD) in erythrocytes of healthy subjects and NIDDM patients after long term administration of 1.0 gm OLE daily for 6 months.

Group	n	MDA (μmol/g Hb)	T- test
Healthy subjects	25	2.22 ± 0.21	
NIDDM patients pre- OLE intake	30	4.44 ± 0.65	P< 0.001
NIDDM patients after- OLE intake	30	2.66 ± 0.33	P< 0.001

Table 3-33. Levels of plasma MDA (Mean ± SD) in healthy and alloxan diabetic rabbits after long term administration of 20 mg OLE daily for 16 weeks.

Group	n	MDA nmol/ml	T- test
Healthy rabbits	8	2.7 ± 0.75	
Alloxan diabetic rabbits pre OLE intake	8	11.5 ± 1.9	P< 0.001
Alloxan diabetic rabbits post OLE intake	8	4.4 ± 0.66	P< 0.001

Table 3-34. Levels of plasma MDA (Mean ± SD) in healthy subjects and NIDDM patients after long term administration of 1.0 gm OLE daily for 6 months

Group	n	MDA nmol/ml	T- test
Healthy subjects	25	3.6 ± 0.75	
NIDDM patients pre- OLE intake	30	28.5 ± 5.5	P< 0.001
NIDDM patients post-OLE intake	30	10.6 ± 3.6	P< 0.001

3.6.12. Effect of OLE intake on erythrocyte SOD activity in alloxan induced diabetic rabbits and NIDDM patient.

The levels of SOD activity in alloxan diabetic rabbit were significantly increased p< 0.001 (0.44 ± 0.08) U/g Hb compared with (0.22 ± 0.05) U/g

Hb in control rabbits, while these levels of SOD activity decrease significantly to (0.25 ± 0.04) U/g Hb in alloxan rabbits receiving 20 mg of OLE daily for 16 week period (Table 3-35).

On the other hand in human study, SOD activity in erythrocyte cells were significantly decreased in NIDDM $(0.32 \pm 0.04$ U/g Hb $)$ compared with control groups $(0.66 \pm 0.05$ U/g Hb$)$, while it was increase in NIDDM receiving 1.0 g OLE daily for 6 months to $(0.42 \pm 0.08$ $)$ as shown in table (3-36).

Subsequent decrease in SOD activity in elderly diabetic suggests that longer disease duration, SOD induction and consequently its activity progressively decrease since no enzymatic later predominates, further hydrogen peroxide has been shown to inhibit Cu/Zn SOD [254] and therefore the accumulation of H_2O_2 caused by the low GPx activity found in NIDDM, could also explain in progressive decrease in SOD in alter stages of the disease.

The decrease of activity of antioxidant enzymatic systems in diabetes is linked to the progressive glycation of enzymatic proteins; about 50% of SOD in erythrocyte cells of diabetic is glycated resulting in trace activity. The increase in peroxide production is believed to be due to insulin deficiency causing chronic metabolic derangement. The increased erythrocyte Cu/Zn SOD activities in alloxan-diabetic rabbits support the hypothesis of radical mediated injury in this disease. Evidence exists that superoxide anion generation measured in serum of type 1 diabetic patients is significantly increased [255]. The primary catalytic cellular defense that protects cells and tissues against potentially destructive reactions of superoxide radicals and their derivatives is the Cu/Zn form of the enzyme. It has also been observed that SOD can be rapidly induced in some conditions when cells or organisms are exposed to oxidative stress [256]. The highest SOD activity in red blood cells found at the onset of diabetes may be interpreted as compensatory activation mechanism due to increased superoxide production, However the marked increase (100%) in the activity of this antioxidant enzyme as shown in table 3-35 at diabetes onset is not sufficient to protect cells during exposure since increased MDA indicates that oxidative cell damage has already occurred.

Table 3-35. Levels of superoxide dismutase activity (Mean ± SD) in erythrocytes of healthy and alloxan diabetic rabbits after long term administration of 20 mg OLE daily for 16 weeks.

Group	n	SOD (U/g Hb)	T- test
Healthy rabbits	8	0.22 ± 0.05	
Alloxan diabetic rabbits pre-OLE intake	8	0.44 ± 0.08	P< 0.001
Alloxan diabetic rabbits post OLE intake	8	0.25 ± 0.04	P< 0.001

Table 3-36. Levels of superoxide dismutase activity (Mean ± SD) in erythrocytes of healthy subjects and NIDDM patients after long term administration of 1.0 gm OLE daily for 6 months.

Group	n	SOD (U/g Hb)	T- test
Healthy subjects	25	0.66 ± 0.05	
NIDDM patients pre-OLE intake	30	0.32 ± 0.04	P< 0.001
NIDDM patients post- OLE intake	30	0.42 ± 0.08	P< 0.001

3.6.13. Effect of OLE intake on erythrocyte catalase activity in alloxan induced diabetic rabbits and NIDDM patients.

From Table 3-37 we obtained that the catalase activity decreased in alloxan diabetic rabbits p<0.05 (0.66 ± 0.12) U/g Hb compared with (1.12 ± 0.3) U/g Hb in control rabbit. After treatment with 20 mg of OLE daily for

16 week period a significant increase in catalase activity was observed which indicated a positive correlation effect of OLE intake. The same results achieved in human study with NIDDM patients as shown in table 3-38. Catalase activity in erythrocyte cells was significantly decreased in NIDDM patients (1.62 ± 0.22) U/ g Hb compared with its activity in healthy subjects (3.12 ± 0.50) U/g Hb, while it increased to (2.11 ± 0.43) U/g Hb in NIDDM patients after long term administration of 1.0 gm OLE daily for 6 months. Our data agree with that reported by Wohaied [124] and in contrast with reported by Dohi [125]. These discrepancies may be partly explained by the variability in the diabetes models used, including the strain and sex of animals, their age at the induction of diabetes, the severity of the resulting insulin deficiency and the duration of diabetes.

Table 3-37. Levels of catalase activity (Mean ± SD) in erythrocytes of healthy and alloxan diabetic rabbits after long term administration of 20 mg OLE daily for 16 weeks.

Group	n	CAT (U/g Hb)	T- test
Healthy rabbits	25	1.12 ± 0.30	
Alloxan diabetic rabbits pre- OLE intake	30	0.66 ± 0.12	P <0.05
Alloxan diabetic rabbits post- OLE intake	30	0.85 ± 0.23	P <0.05

Table 3-38. Levels of catalase activity (Mean ± SD) in erythrocytes of healthy subjects and NIDDM patients after long term administration of 1.0 gm OLE daily for 6 months.

Group	n	CAT (U/g Hb)	T- test
Healthy subjects	25	3.12 ± 0.50	
NIDDM patients pre- OLE intake	30	1.62 ± 0.22	P < 0.05
NIDDM patients post- OLE intake	30	2.11 ± 0.43	P < 0.05

3.6.14. Effect of OLE intake on erythrocyte glucose 6-PD activity in alloxan induced diabetic rabbit and NIDDM patients.

A significant decrease in the G-6PD activity had been obtained in alloxan diabetic rabbits P <0.05 (0.55 ± 0.25) U/g Hb as compared with (1.5 ± 0.32) U/g Hb in non diabetic rabbit while the activity of G-6PD increased to (1.1 ± 0.28) U/g Hb when the alloxan diabetic rabbit receiving 20 mg of OLE daily for 16 week period (table 3-39). The positive effect of OLE intake by alloxan induced diabetic rabbits not only normalized blood glucose levels in a manner similar to insulin but also positively affected the expression of G-6PD a key metabolic enzyme, our data confirmed with that reported by Berg [257].

Treatment of the diabetic animals with OLE restored the activity of G-6PD activity to about 80-90% of their normal values. The main biological function of G-6PD is to support reductive biosynthesis as well as to maintain an environment in the tissue, thereby preventing free radical induced complication leading to cataract formation and other secondary complication of diabetes [258]. On the other hand in human study the same results were obtained as shown in table (3-40).

The levels of G-6PD activity significantly reduced in NIDDM patients $p < 0.001$ (3.3 ± 1.3) U/g Hb compared with (7.5 ± 1.2) U/g Hb in healthy subjects, while these levels raised to (6.6 ± 1.4) U/g Hb in NIDDM patients receiving 1.0 gm of OLE daily for 6 month period.

The results of this study were in consistent with that reported by Berg [257]. Here as we demonstrated previously OLE is an active ingredient in olive leaf extract had a good power of antioxidant against free radicals and other reactive species that injury tissue in diabetic patients. Intake OLE daily leads to increase total antioxidant status and improvement the glycemic control and antioxidant enzyme activity as well as the non enzymatic antioxidant like vitamin E and C retained in levels near the borderline of healthy condition.

Table 3-39. Levels of erythrocyte G-6PD activity (Mean ± SD) in healthy and alloxan diabetic rabbits after long term administration of 20mg OLE daily for 16 weeks.

Group	n	G-6PD (U/g Hb)	T- test
Healthy rabbits	8	1.5 ± 0.32	
Alloxan diabetic rabbits pre-OLE intake	8	0.55 ± 0.25	P<0.05
Alloxan diabetic rabbits post-OLE intake	8	1.1 ± 0.28	P<0.05

Table 3-40. Levels of erythrocyte G-6PD activity (Mean ± SD) in healthy subjects and NIDDM patients after long term administration of 1.0 gm OLE daily for 6 months.

Group	n	G-6PD (U/g Hb)	T- test
Healthy subjects	25	7.5 ±1.2	
NIDDM patients pre- OLE intake	30	3.3 ± 1.3	P<0001
NIDDM patients post- OLE intake	30	6.6 ±1.4	P<0001

3.6.15. Effect of OLE intake on plasma and erythrocyte GSH levels in alloxan induced diabetic rabbits and NIDDM patients.

GSH content in erythrocyte of alloxan diabetic rabbits was determined as shown in table (3-41).There was a significant decrease $P < 0.05$ (2.25 ± 0.30) µmol/g Hb compared with (4.55 ± 0.5)) µmol/g Hb in control rabbits, while these levels increased significantly to (3.95 ± 0.45) µmol/g Hb in alloxan diabetic rabbits receiving 20 mg of OLE daily for 16 week period, in addition to, the GSH content in plasma of alloxan diabetic rabbits was also decreased (0.55 ± 0.25) µmol/ml compared with (1.50 ± 0.32) µmol/ml in control rabbits and after OLE intake the GSH content increased to (1.1 ± 0.28) µmol/ ml) as shown in table (3-43).

Table(3-42) showed that GSH content in erythrocytes of NIDDM patients was significantly lower in NIDDM patients (6.5 ± 0.45 µmol/g Hb) compared with the levels of the control subjects (11.3 ± 0.66 µmol/g Hb) p<0.05, while it was increased in NIDDM patients receiving 1.0 gm of OLE daily for 6 months to (9.9 ± 0.43) µmol/g Hb. On the other hand we obtained the same pattern of data when we determined the GSH content in plasma NIDDM patients before and after OLE intake as shown in table (3-44) consistent with the findings of other investigators in type one and two diabetic adults suggesting that GSH metabolism is altered in both types [258-259].

Several studies support the hypothesis that in diabetes chronic hyperglycemia increases the polyol pathway, as well as AGE formation and free radical generation rates, which lead to increased GSH oxidation [260-261]. A relative depletion of NADPH due to aldose reductase activation and secondary to reduced production through the pentose cycle impairs GSH regeneration and leads to depletion of this free radical scavenger. GSH the most prevalent low molecular weight peptide antioxidant in cells participate in many cellular functions including detoxification process such as protection of the SH group of cystiene in proteins and elimination of hydrogen peroxide (GSH redox cycle) by direct interaction with free radicals and regeneration of oxidized vitamin E [262-263].

Therefore, changes in GSH redox status could be considered a particularly sensitive indicator of oxidative stress. Intake of OLE by diabetic patients IDDM and NIDDM had been given an indication of improvement a hyperglycemia status and oxidative stress, through improvement of antioxidant enzyme activity and retain the balance between oxidant / antioxidant ratio similar that in normal healthy subject [258].

Table 3-41. Levels of GSH (Mean ± SD) in erythrocytes of healthy and alloxan diabetic rabbits after long term administration of 20 mg oleuropein daily after 16 weeks.

Group	n	GSH (µmol/g Hb)	T- test
Healthy rabbits	8	4.55 ± 0.50	
Alloxan diabetic rabbits pre-OLE intake	8	2.25 ± 0.30	P< 0.001
Alloxan diabetic rabbits post- OLE intake	8	3.95 ± 0.45	P < 0.05

Table 3-42. Levels of GSH (Mean ± SD) in erythrocytes of healthy subjects and NIDDM patients after long term administration of 1.0 gm oleuropein daily after 6 months.

Group	n	GSH (µmol/g Hb)	T- test
Healthy subjects	25	11.2 ± 0.66	
NIDDM patients pre- OLE intake	30	6.2 ± 0.45	P< 0.001
NIDDM patients post- OLE intake	30	9.9 ± 0.43	P < 0.05

Table 3-43. Levels of plasma GSH (Mean ± SD) in healthy and alloxan diabetic rabbits after long term administration of 20 mg OLE daily for 16 weeks.

Group	n	GSH (µmol/ml	T- test
Healthy rabbits	8	1.5 ± 0.32	
Alloxan diabetic rabbits pre-OLE intake	8	0.55 ± 0.25	P < 0.05
Alloxan diabetic rabbits post-OLE intake	8	1.1 ± 0.28	P < 0.05

Table 3-44. Levels of plasma GSH (Mean ± SD) in healthy subjects and NIDDM patients after long term administration of 1.0 gm OLE daily for 6 months.

Group	n	GSH (µmol/ml	T- test
Healthy subjects	25	7.5 ± 2.2	
NIDDM patients pre- OLE intake	30	5.0 ± 2.5	P < 0.05
NIDDM patients post- OLE intake	30	6.6 ± 2.4	P < 0.05

3.6.16. Effect of OLE intake on erythrocyte glutathione peroxidase activity in alloxan induced diabetic rabbits and NIDDM patients.

From table (3-45) the result had been shown that there was a significant decrease in glutathione peroxidase activity in alloxan diabetic rabbits $p<0.001$ (7.55 ± 1.9) U/g Hb compared with (12.5 ± 2.5) U/g Hb in non diabetic rabbits, while a significant increase in the activity of GPx (10.5 ± 1.7) U/g Hb obtained after alloxan diabetic rabbits receiving 20 mg of OLE daily for 16 week period. Erythrocyte GPx activity was lower in NIDDM patients(18.7 ± 7.7 U/g Hb) compared with control group (27.3 ± 5.3 U/g Hb), while it was increased in NIDDM receiving OLE 1.0 gm daily for 6 months to (24.5 ± 3.6) as shown in table (3-46).

The results demonstrated that erythrocyte GPx activity was significantly lower in NIDDM patients compared with control groups that agreed with those of Jos et al, the low GPx activity could be directly explained by the low GSH content found in NIDDM patients, since GSH is a substrate and cofactor of this enzyme. Therefore low GSH content implies low GPx activity which may produce increased oxidative stress, enzymatic inactivation could also contribute to low Gpx activity, *in vitro* studies have been shown that although Gpx is a relatively stable enzyme, it may be inactivated under conditions of severe oxidative stress [264].

Carmen D. et al showed that enzymatic inactivation might occur through glycation governed by prevailing glucose concentration thus increased glycation in diabetic patients and the subsequent reactions of proteins might affect amino acids close to the active sites of the molecule or disturb the sterochemical configuration thereby provoking structural and functional changes in protein [265].

On the other hand results showed a possible disarrangement between high enzymatic SOD activity and low Gpx activity in erythrocytes of diabetic patients. Because Gpx removes hydrogen peroxide produced by the SOD catalyzed reaction an imbalance between the two enzymes may occur. In fact activities of both antioxidant enzymes in the control were positively correlated. In contrast, this correlation in the diabetic group was not maintained which suggests that the functional relationship was disrupted and therefore possibly harmful to cells.

Table 3-45. Levels of glutathione peroxidase activity (Mean ± SD) in erythrocytes of healthy and alloxan diabetic rabbits after long term administration of 20 mg OLE daily after 16 weeks.

Group	n	GPx (U/g Hb)	T- test
Healthy rabbits	8	12.5 ± 2.5	
Alloxan diabetic rabbits pre-OLE intake	8	7.55 ± 1.9	P< 0.001
Alloxan diabetic rabbits post-OLE intake	8	10.5 ± 1.7	P <0.001

Table 3-46. Levels of glutathione peroxidase activity (Mean ± SD) in erythrocytes of healthy subjects and NIDDM patients after long term administration of 1.0 gm OLE daily after 6 months.

Group	n	GPx (U/g Hb)	T- test
Healthy subjects	25	27.3 ± 5.3	
NIDDM patients pre-OLE intake	30	18.7 ± 7.7	P <0.001
NIDDM patients post -OLE intake	30	24.5 ±3.6	P <0.001

3.6.17. Effect of OLE intake on erythrocyte glutathione reductase activity in alloxan induced diabetic rabbits and NIDDM patients.

From table (3-47) a significant decrease in erythrocyte glutathione reductase activity was observed in alloxan induced diabetic rabbits $p<0.05$ (2.7 ± 0.25) U/g Hb compared with (4.4 ± 0.27) U/g Hb in control rabbits while it was increased to (3.5 ± 0.32) U/ g Hb levels after receiving 20 mg daily of OLE for 16 weeks. The same results in animal study were noticed in human study, the activity of GRx in NIDDM patients was reduced to (6.0 ± 0.75) U/g Hb compared with (8.5 ± 0.25) U/g Hb in healthy subjects. After a long treatment by 1.0 gm OLE for 6 months the activity of GRx is increased to (7.6 ± 0.45) U/ g Hb due to OLE positive effect (Table 3-48).

Table 3-47. Levels of glutathione reductase activity (Mean ± SD) in erythrocytes of healthy and alloxan diabetic rabbits after long term administration of 20 mg OLE daily for 16 weeks.

Group	n	GRx (U/g Hb	T- test
Healthy rabbits	8	4.4 ± 0.27	
Alloxan diabetic rabbits pre-OLE intake	8	2.7 ± 0.25	P<0.05
Alloxan diabetic rabbits post-OLE intake	8	3.5 ± 0.32	P<0.05

Table 3-48. Levels of glutathione reductase activity (Mean ± SD) in erythrocytes of healthy subjects and NIDDM patients after long term administration of 1.0 gm OLE daily for 6 month.

Group	n	GRx (U/g Hb)	T- test
Healthy subjects	25	8.5 ± 0.25	
NIDDM patients pre-OLE intake	30	6.0 ± 0.75	P < 0.05
NIDDM patients post- OLE intake	30	7.6 ± 0.45	P < 0.05

3.8.18. Effect of OLE intake on serum vit. E levels in alloxan induced diabetic rabbits and NIDDM patients

There was a significant decrease in the levels of vitamin E in alloxan diabetic rabbit p<0.05 (0.26 ± 0.10) mg/dl compared with (0.55 ± 0.15) mg/dl in non diabetic control rabbits, while these values increased significantly p<0.05 to (0.40 ± 0.20) mg/dl in alloxan diabetic rabbits receiving 20 mg of OLE daily for 16 week period (Table 3-49).

Plasma α-tocopherol concentrations were significantly lower in NIDDM patients (0.75±0.2) mg/dl compared with healthy subjects (1.55 ± 0.72) mg/dl as shown in table (3-50). The reason of reducing levels of vit. E in NIDDM patients may be due to many factors: first glucophage affect the absorption process of nutrient food, second hyperglycemia state in NIDDM patients play an important role in increased production of MDA, lipid per-oxidation, increased oxidized LDL levels so loss of antioxidant such as vit E is expected. When patients with NIDDM intake OLE 1.0 gm daily for 6 months, the levels of vit. E are increased to the same level as in healthy control group(1.22 ± 0.25) mg/dl, due to influence of OLE in improvement blood glucose levels, increased in total antioxidant capacity, inhibition of lipid per-oxidation process and reduced levels of MDA.   Extra cellular fluids contain non-enzymatic antioxidant that may delay or inhibit the oxidative process [265].

Enhanced lipid per-oxidation increases the need for lipid soluble antioxidant such as vit. E and β-carotene thus, plasma vit. E levels in the NIDDM patients were less than from those of control group. Nevertheless when the values were normalized by total lipids, low ratios in NIDDM patients were found, changes after lipid correction were probably due to insulin-glucagon imbalances in diabetic patients, which lead to elevated plasma lipid levels with increased triglycerides and cholesterol [266]. Tocopherol is the primary *in vivo* chain breaking, lipid soluble antioxidant in human serum and is particularly effective in lipid per-oxidation inhibition so OLE intake increase the total antioxidant status, alternatively the levels of vit. E keeps in baseline levels as in healthy subjects [267].

Table 3-49. Levels of vitamin E (Mean ± SD) in healthy and alloxan diabetic rabbits after long term administration of 20 mg OLE daily for 16 weeks.

Group	n	Vit E (mg/dl)	T- test
Healthy rabbits	8	0.55 ± 0.15	
Alloxan diabetic rabbits pre-OLE intake	8	0.26 ± 0.10	P < 0.05
Alloxan diabetic rabbits post-OLE intake	8	0.40 ± 0.20	P < 0.05

Table 3-50. Levels of vitamin E (Mean ± SD) in healthy subjects and NIDDM after long term administration of 1.0 gm OLE daily for 6 months.

Group	n	Vit E (mg/dl)	T- test
Healthy subjects	25	1.55 ± 0.75	
NIDDM patients pre- OLE intake	30	0.76 ± 0.20	P < 0.05
NIDDM patients post-OLE intake	30	1.22 ± 0.25	P < 0.05

3.6.19. Effect of OLE intake on serum vitamin C levels in alloxan diabetic rabbits and NIDDM patients.

The levels of vitamin C were significantly decreased in alloxan diabetic rabbits p<0.05(0.20 ±0.13) mg/dl Vs. (0.45 ± 0.12) mg/dl in control rabbits, while these levels increased significantly p<0.05 (0.35 ± 0.10) mg/dl in alloxan diabetic rabbit receiving 20 mg of OLE daily for 16 week period, as shown in table (3-51).

On the other hand, a significant decrease of levels of vitamin C in NIDDM patients is observed compared with healthy subjects (0.75 ± 0.33 Vs. 1.55 ± 0.22) mg/dl respectively, while it increased to 1.22 ± 0.30 mg/dl in NIDDM patients whom receiving 1.0 gm OLE daily for 6 months (table 3-52).

Our results are agree well with pervious studies which suggests that persons with diabetes mellitus have lower circulating vitamin C concentrations than those without this disorder, [268] this is indeed true, this deficit in persons with diabetes may be one factor contributing to their increased risk of infection, damage to connective tissue, and oxidative tissue damage[269].Several explanations for reduced serum vitamin C concentrations in persons with diabetes might be considered to (1) renal reabsorption of vitamin C may be reduced by hyperglycemia, (2) blood glucose may compete with vitamin C for uptake into certain cells and tissues, (3) cellular regulation of vitamin C may be impaired, and (4) increased oxidative stress may deplete antioxidant reserves [268].

Lower vitamin C levels observed in patients with NIDDM may be increased to normal baseline after OLE intake due to the positive effect of OLE in improvement glycemic condition, increase the total antioxidant statue, increased blood flow and a consequence to this positive effect levels of vitamin C become near normal in NIDDM patients.

Table 3-51. Levels of vitamin C (Mean ± SD) in healthy and alloxan diabetic rabbits after long term administration of 20 mg OLE daily for 16 weeks.

Group	n	Vit. C (mg/dl)	T- test
Healthy rabbits	8	0.45 ± 0.12	
Alloxan diabetic rabbits pre- OLE intake	8	0.20 ± 0.13	P< 0.05
Alloxan diabetic rabbits post- OLE intake	8	0.35 ± 0.10	P< 0.05

Table 3-52. Levels of vitamin C (Mean ± SD) in healthy subjects and NIDDM patients after long term administration of 1.0 gm OLE daily for 6 months.

Group	n	Vit.C (mg/dl)	T- test
Healthy subjects	25	1.55 ± 0.22	
NIDDM patients pre- OLE intake	30	0.75 ± 0.33	P< 0.05
NIDDM patients post- OLE intake	30	1.22 ± 0.30	P< 0.05

3.6.20. Effect of OLE intake on plasma β-carotene levels in alloxan induced diabetic rabbits and NIDDM patients.

Table (3-53) showed that the levels of β--carotene in alloxan diabetic rabbits were significantly decreased p < 0.001 (0.14 ± 0.02) μmol/L compared with (0.33 ± 0.03) μmol/L in control rabbits, while these levels were increased to (0.26 ± 0.04) μmol/L in alloxan diabetic rabbits receiving 20 mg of OLE daily for 16 week period. Plasma levels of β -carotene were significantly lower in NIDDM patients (0.35 ± 0.07) μmole/L than in control subjects (0.75 ± 0.09) μmol/L, and these values were increased to (0.55 ± 0.08) μmol/L after OLE intake by NIDDM patients for 6 months as a shown in table (3-54). β -carotene, also a lipid soluble and chain breaking antioxidant, is an effective quencher of singlet oxygen and can inhibit lipid per-oxidation, exhibiting effective radical trapping antioxidant behavior only at low physiological oxygen pressures [270].

The difference in plasma concentrations between NIDDM patients and healthy control groups may be due to rapid turnover of β -carotene, perhaps through quenching of oxygen radicals since β-carotene is consumed faster than alpha-tocopherol when the radicals are generated within the lipophilic compartment of the membranes [271].

The findings suggest a therapeutic role for antioxidant in protection islets from oxidative damage by free radicals in the pre-diabetic period of the disease, treatment with OLE which is proved a potent antioxidant than vit. E might reduce the per-oxidation rate, restore the body antioxidant capacity and possibly prevent or delay development of type 1 diabetes especially in subjects immunologically identified to be at high risk for developing IDDM.

Table 3-53. Levels of plasma β -carotene (Mean ± SD) in healthy and alloxan diabetic rabbits after long term administration of 20 mg OLE daily for 16 weeks.

Group	n	Carotene µmol/1	T- test
Healthy rabbits	8	0.33 ± 0.03	
Alloxan diabetic rabbits pre- OLE intake	8	0.14 ± 0.02	P< 0.001
Alloxan diabetic rabbits Post-OLE intake	8	0.26 ± 0.04	P<0.05

Table 3-54. Levels of plasma β-carotene (Mean ± SD) in healthy subjects and NIDDM patients after long term administration of 1.0 gm OLE daily for 6 months.

Group	n	Carotene (µmol/L)	T- test
Healthy subjects	25	0.75 ± 0.09	
NIDDM patients pre-OLE intake	30	0.35 ±0.07	P< 0.001
NIDDM patients post-OLE intake	30	0.55 ± 0.08	P< 0.05

3.6.21. Effect of OLE intake on serum total antioxidant capacity (TEAC) in alloxan induced diabetic rabbits and NIDDM patients.

The results of this study demonstrated that the antioxidant capacity of animal or human serum measured as TEAC was increased over the end of the study. From table (3-55) a significant increase was observed for TEAC in alloxan induced rabbits after along term administration of 20 mg oleuropein daily (220 ± 26 µmol/L) compared with diabetic rabbit before treatment (133 ± 25 µmol/L). The same results had been obtained in NIDDM patients as showed in table (3-56). These results suggest the role of oleuropein in its antioxidant property in substitution the lack of total antioxidant which had been occurred in diabetes disease, since oleuropein may be acting locally to protect other dietary antioxidants such vitamin C and E from degradation in the intestine, this would contribute to a beneficial increase in the total antioxidant status of the body by enhancing the bioavailability of the other dietary antioxidant. On the other hand these results suggest that the total antioxidant capacity of serum is part of a tightly regulated homeostatic mechanism, this was expected because an efficient antioxidant defense is important in the control of oxidative stress caused by free radicals and other reactive species, which are continuously generated in the body [272].

Table 3-55. Levels of serum total antioxidant capacity (Mean ± SD) in healthy and alloxan diabetic rabbits after long term administration of 20 mg OLE daily for 6 weeks.

Group	n	TEAC (µmol/L)	T-test
Healthy rabbits	8	250 ± 22	
Alloxan diabetic rabbits pre-OLE intake	8	133 ± 25	P < 0.001
Alloxan diabetic rabbits post-OLE intake	8	220 ± 26	P < 0.001

Table 3-56. Levels of serum total antioxidant capacity (Mean ± SD) in healthy subjects and NIDDM patients after long term administration of 1.0 gm OLE daily for 6 months.

Group	n	TEAC (µmol/L)	T-test
Healthy subjects	25	420 ± 42	
NIDDM patients pre OLE-intake	30	210 ± 37	P< 0.001
NIDDM patients post OLE-intake	30	380 ± 35	P< 0.001

3.7. Toxicity of crude oleuropein

The safety limits of polyphenolic compound (crude oleuropein) isolated from olive leaves was recognized by measuring the activities of alanine aminotransferase(GPT), aspatrate aminotransferase (GOT), alkaline phosphatase (ALP), total serum bilirubin, blood urea , serum creatinine, serum albumin and total protein, in healthy rabbits supplemented up to 5.0 gm daily of crude oleuropein for 16 week period. The results of biochemical assays had been shown no significant change against control rabbits (without supplemented oleuropein.

Oleuropein has undergone extensive toxicological testing and has produced no adverse effects when given in large doses to animals under study over long periods of time. The only adverse effect of using olive leaf extract to fight off an active infection is a counter response known as the Herxheimer reaction. The body's own immune system destroys the dead bacteria and the breakdown products can cause a variety of toxic symptoms. Some detoxification symptoms may occur with the initial use of OLE as it kills bad microbes faster than the body can eliminate them. This is easily remedied by reducing the dosage for a few days to allow the animal's waste disposal system to catch up once the cleaning takes place, which may take up to several days, energy levels will increase and the symptoms will subside[273-274].

3.8. Microbiology Studies

3.8.1. Effect of oleuropein on bacterial growth and determination of MIC

Initial screening of potential antibacterial and antifungal compounds from plants may be performed with pure substances or crude extracts. The methods used for the two types of organisms are similar. The two most commonly used to determine antimicrobial susceptibility are the broth dilution assay and the disc or agar well diffusion assay. Clinical microbiologists are very familiar with these assays, at this stage, more specific media can be used and MICs can be effectively compared to those of a wider range of currently used antibiotics. The investigation of olive leaves extract effective against many resistant bacteria provides an example of prospecting for new compounds which may be particularly effective against infections that are currently difficult to treat with available antibiotics.

Oleuropein one of the major classes of polyphenol contained in olives have recently shown to inhibit or delay the rate of growth of a range of bacteria but there are no data in the literature concerning the possible employment of these polyphenolic secoiridoids as antimicrobial agents against pathogenic bacteria in man. In this study five standard strains (*Haemophilus influenzae* ATCC 9006, *Salmonella typhi* ATCC 6539, *Staphylococcus aureus* ATCC 25923, *E.coli* ATCC 7200, and *Klebsiella Pneumonia* ATCC 6645 and ten fresh clinical isolates (*Salmonella typhi.* 2 strains, *Staphylococcus aureus* 2 strains *E.coli* 2 strains, *Klebseilla Pneumonia* 2 strains ,and *Haemophilus influenzae* 2 strains were used.These causal agents of intestinal or respiratory tract and UTI infections were tested for in vitro susceptibility to oleuropein, oleuropein aglycone, hydroxytyrosol and elenolic acid.

From results in figure (3-11) oleuropein had no effect on all species of bacteria either standard or locally isolated strains at any concentration used (25, 50, 100, 200, and 300 µg/ml), while oleuropein aglycone showed a positive effect in all species under study at a concentration of 100 µg/ml. The range of diameter inhibition zones were 28 mm for *E.coli*, 24 mm for *K.pneumonia,* 20 mm for *salmonella.typhi,* 18 mm for *H.influnenza* and 17 mm for *staph. aureus* species.

The antimicrobial activity of oleuropein metabolite: oleuropein aglycone, hydroxytyrosol and elenolic acid against different bacterial species used in this study ordered as follow:

Oleuropein aglycone > hydroxytyrosol> elenolic acid

The sensitivity of different bacterial species against the oleuropein metabolite ordered as follow:

E.coli > Klebseilla Pneumonia > Salmonella typhi. > Haemophilus influenza > Staphylococcus aureus

The minimum inhibitory concentrations (MICs) are evidence for the broad antimicrobial activity of oleuropein aglycone against all those bacterial strains (MIC values between 40-110 µg/ml for standard strains and between 75-130 µg/ml for clinical isolated strains table (3-57& 58). These data indicate that in addition to the potential employment of its active principles as food additives, *Olea europeae* can be considered a potential source of promising antimicrobial agents for treatment of intestinal or respiratory, and urinary tract infection in man. The maximum bactericidal concentration was twice value of the minimum inhibitory concentration in all bacterial strains as shown in table(3-59, 3-60), which may be related to genetic factors.

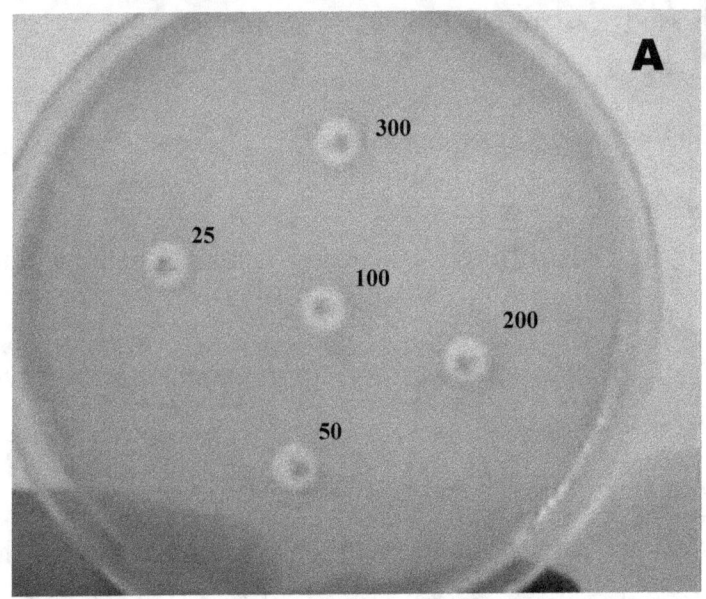

Figure 3-11. Antimicrobial activity of oleuropein (OLE) and its metabolites: oleuropein aglycone (OLEa), Hydroxytyrosol (HT), and Elenolic acid (EA) on different species of pathogenic bacteria .**A.** Effect of Different (25, 50, 100, 200 and 300 µg/ml) on growth of *E.coli.*

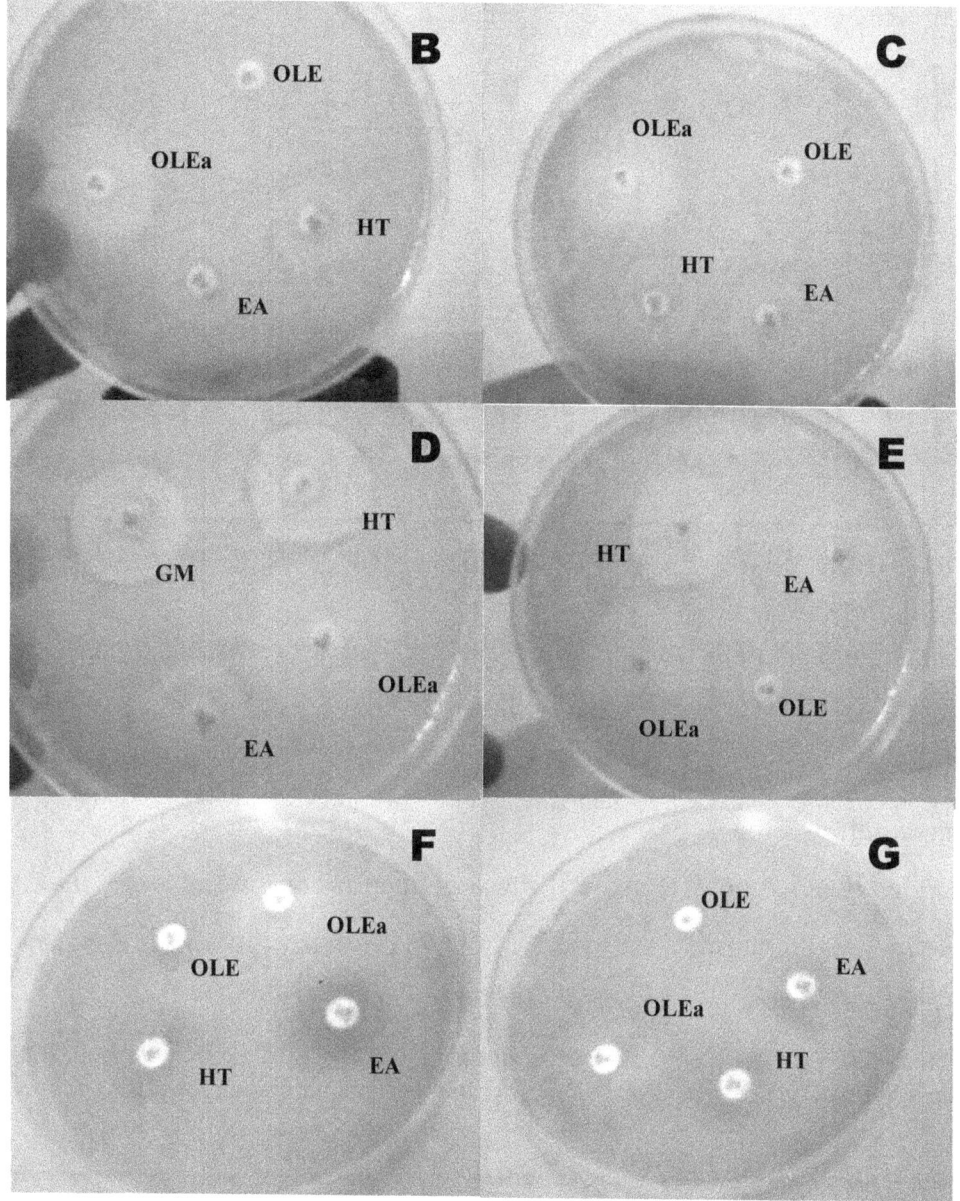

Figure 3-11 Continued.

B: Effect of OLE and its metabolite on *Salmonella typhi*.

C: Effect of OLE and its metabolites on *H.influenza*.

D: Effect of OLE and its metabolites on *E.coli*.

E: Effect of OLE and its metabolite on *K.pneumonia*.

F: Effect of OLE and its metabolite on *Staph.aureus*

G: Effect of OLE and its metabolites on *Staph. aureus* (standard strain).

* GM = Gentamicin antibiotic(30 µg/ml) used or comparison.

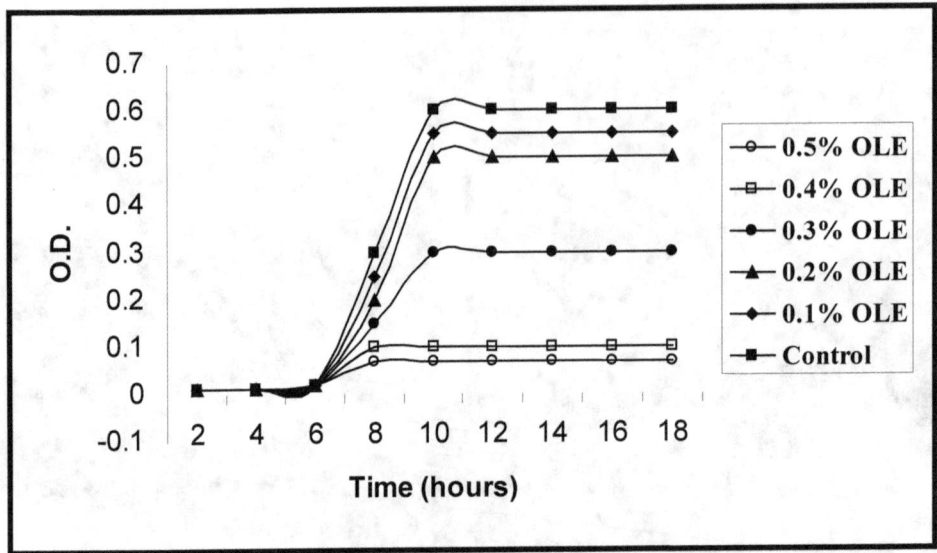

Figure 3-12. The effect of different concentration of OLEa on growth of *staph.aureus*

From Figure (3-12) oleuropein aglycone 0.1% (w/v) was observed to delay growth of *staph.aureus* in the lag phase, (0.3 % w/v) of oleuropein aglycone inhibited 50% of growth of *staph.aureus* at the lag phase, while at a concentration (0.4% w/v) the growth of *staph aureus* was inhibited completely since no effect of all these concentration on the *staph.aureus* at the exponential phase.

Table 3-57. The MIC (µg/ ml) of oleuropein (OLE); oleuropein aglycone (OLEa); hydroxytyrosol (HT) and elenolic acid (EA) to some standard strain of different bacterial species.

Standard strains	OLE	OLEa	HT	EA
H.influenza ATCC 9006,	---	100	110	134
S.aureus ATCC 25923	---	110	125	144
Salm.Typhi ATCC 6539	---	90	100	115
E.coli ATCC 7200	---	40	50	50
K.pneumonia ATCC 6645	---	75	85	95

Table 3-58. The MIC (µg /ml) of oleuropein (OLE); oleuropein aglycone, hydroxytyrosol (HT) and elenolic acid (EA) to some clinical isolate strains of different bacteria species.

Locally clinical isolates	OLE	OLEa	HT	EA
H.influenza	---	120	140	150
S.auerus	---	130	150	1160
Salm.Typhi	---	100	125	140
E.coli	---	75	90	100
K.pneumonia	---	100	110	125

Table 3-59. The MBC (µg/ml) of oleuropein (OLE); oleuropein aglycone (OLEa); hydroxytyrosol (HT) and elenolic acid (EA) to some standard strain of different bacterial species.

Standard strains	OLE	OLEa	HT	EA
H.influenza ATCC 9006,	---	200	220	270
S.aureus ATCC 25923	---	220	250	280
Salm.Typhi ATCC 6539	---	180	200	230
E.coli ATCC 7200	---	80	100	100
K.pneumonia ATCC 6645	---	150	170	180

Table 3-60. The MBC (µg/ml) of oleuropein (OLE); oleuropein aglycone, hydroxytyrosol (HT) and elenolic acid (EA) to some clinical isolate strains of different bacteria species.

Locally clinical isolates	OLE	OLEa	HT	EA
H.influenza	---	240	280	300
S.auerus	---	260	300	320
Salm.Typhi	---	200	250	300
E.coli	---	150	180	200
K.pneumonia	---	200	220	250

Oleuropein the bitter principle of olive leaves inhibits the growth of various bacteria under study. Its structure is that of a phenolic glycoside according to Foggs [275]. The antimicrobial action of phenols is related to their ability to denature proteins and they are generally classified among the surface active agents, they act by causing leakage of cytoplasmic constituents of the bacterial cells, resulting from damage to the cell membrane affecting its permeability. Phenolic disinfectants at sub lethal concentration cause an increase in the leakage of cell constituents of inorganic phosphate from E coli, glutamic acid and potassium from cells of L. plantarum, leakage could be due to a mechanical injury as well as damage of regulatory mechanisms controlling permeability of the cell membrane [276].

OLE had no influence on the rate of glycolsis, so OLE does not affect the activity of the glycoltic enzymes [275]. The mode of antibacterial action of OLE is similar to that of other phenolic compounds and surface active substances; however it seems that OLE is more selective than simple phenol as seen from the heterogeneity in the sensitivity of different bacteria to OLE. The presence of antimicrobial compounds in olives has been suspected for some time. Flemening et al (1973) and Walter et al (1973) reported the antimicrobial activity of oleuropein and its enzymatic hydrolysis product against bacteria and yeast, however not enough data were available to identify the chemical structure of the enzymatic degradation product, nor could be they examine the antimicrobial activity of the pure compound [37,277].

The activity of oleuropein is due to the aglycone hemiacetal or the corresponding aglycone cleaved enol-aldehyde structure. The strong activity of oleuropein could be caused by the alpha-beta unsaturated aldehyde structure. Double bonds in the alpha-beta unsaturated carbonyl structure were known to react with nucleophilic as in the case of drimane type dialdhyde sesquiterepnes and sesquiterepnes lactones [278], also it has been observed that the double bond stabilizes a bond formed between an aldehyde and an amino residue [279] .The fact that oleuropein is a secoiridoid glycoside without a cyclopentane ring could be another reason for the strong activity of oleuropein .Iridoid aglycone are supposed to be in equilibrium between an open ring glutaraldehyde like structure and a closed ring structure, in theory the open ring structure of oleuropein aglycone can rotate around two axes whereas the open ring structures of genipin and aucubin can rotate around only one. The free movement around two axes might favor the open ring structure in equilibrium which is an active form [280].

Figure (3-13). The chemical structure of the active part corresponding to antimicrobial activity in oleuropein.

3.9. Radioreceptor studies

3.9.1. Effect of different cell concentration on I^{125}-insulin binding to human lymphocyte

To determine whether the different cell concentration of lymphocyte cells effect the binding of I^{125}-insulin, increasing amounts of cell concentration were incubated with labeled insulin for 75 minutes at 15C°, in the presence of $(5\times10^{-11}M)$ I^{125}-insulin. In each experiment, cells over the entire concentration range were incubated with labeled insulin in the presence of $(8\times10^{-8} M)$ unlabeled insulin .Radioactivity bound to the cells under these conditions was considered "non-specific binding (NSB)" and

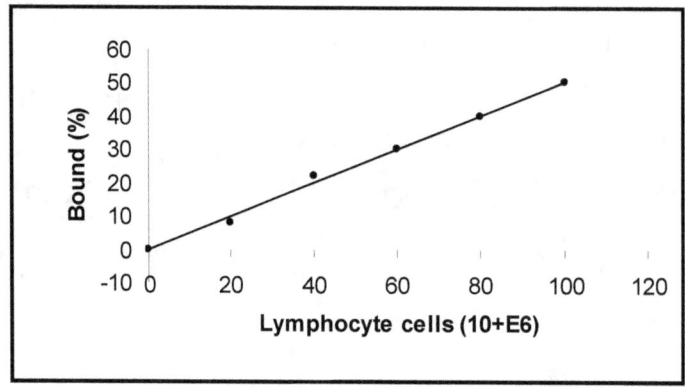

Figure 3-14. Effect of lymphocyte cells concentration on I^{125}-insulin binding to human lymphocytes. Peripheral lymphocytes from normal subjects were incubated for 75 min at 15 C° in the presence of 5 x 10^{-11} M of labeled insulin. In each experiment, cells over the entire concentration range were incubated with labeled insulin in the presence of 8 x 10^{-8}M unlabelled insulin Radioactivity bound to the cells under these conditions was considered non- specific binding and these values were subtracted from each point to correct for the contribution of the nonspecific to the total binding.

these values were subtracted from each point to correct for the concentration of the NSB to total binding. Figure (3-14) shows the increasing values of (%B) with increasing amount of cell concentration of the lymphocyte cell isolated from NIDDM patients, so the binding of labeled insulin is a function of the cell concentration. There is a linear increase in the (%B) over a 50 fold increase in cell concentration.

3.9.2. Effect of time on the binding of I^{125}-insulin with lymphocyte cells isolated from NIDDM patients.

To choose the most appropriate incubation time at (4 C°, 15 C°, 37 C° and 45 C°) the experiment was carried out at different time intervals (5-100 min). Figure (3-15) shows that the optimum binding of labeled insulin to the binding sites in lymphocyte cells isolated from NIDDM patients was occurred at 60 min.

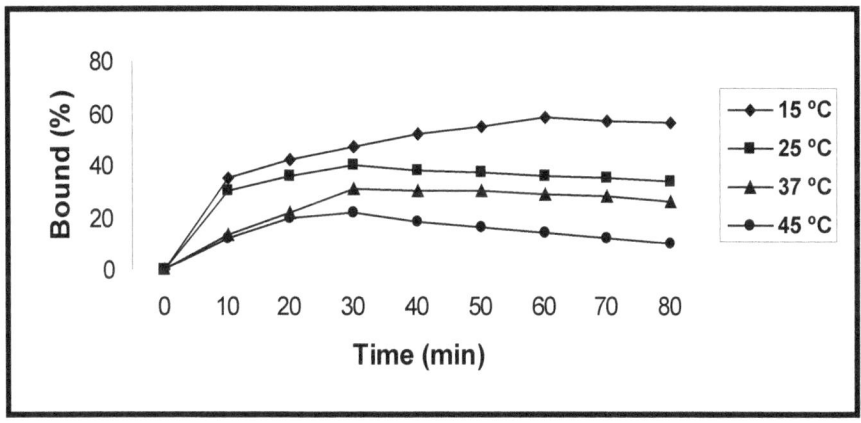

Figure 3-15. I^{125}-insulin binding to peripheral human lymphocytes as a function of time and temperature. Cells (1 ×10^8 cell/ml) were incubated with 1×10^{-11} M labeled insulin. Points have been corrected for nonspecific binding.

3.9.3. Effect of temperature on the binding of I^{125}-insulin with lymphocyte cells isolated from NIDDM patients

The temperature dependency of the binding of I^{125}-insulin to the lymphocyte cell isolated from NIDDM patients was investigated. Figure (3-15) reveals that the binding of labeled insulin to its receptor on the membrane of lymphocyte cells decreased when the temperature was raised due to released surface insulin binding molecules into the medium or may be due to the irreversible dissociation of the insulin-receptor complex or the loss of binding activity may be due to degradation of insulin, according to these results, 15C° was used in all the further experiments for binding kinetics studied.

3.9.4. Effect of different pH on the binding of I^{125}-insulin with the lymphocyte cells isolated from NIDDM patients

The analysis of the influence of pH on binding of labeled insulin with the lymphocyte cells isolated from NIDDM patients was shown in figure (3-16) the optimum pH was found to be 7.8 for NIDDM patients. The same figure showed a decreasing in the binding percent bound/total at the pH higher or lower than the optimum pH. These results indicate that the shift in the pH of the medium may affect the properties of the macromolecules involved in the binding. This effect includes the induction of protonation-deprotonation process occurring within the ionizable groups of amino groups present in the binding domain of these membrane receptors. According to the results obtained in this experiment the pH of incubation buffer in all subsequent was adjusted at 7.8 as optimum pH for all next binding studies.

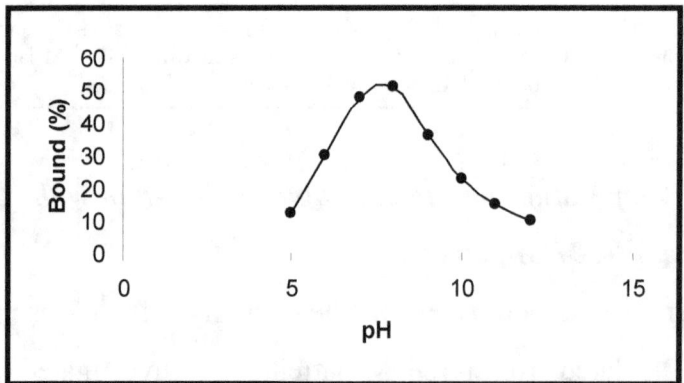

Figure (3-16). Effect of pH on specific binding of labeled insulin (I-125) with human lymphocytes

3.9.5. Kinetic studies

The binding of I^{125}-insulin to the lymphocyte receptor is time and temperature dependent maximum binding occurs at 15 C°, a steady state is reached by 60 min and maintained for at least one hour. At 25C° and 37C° the maximal binding is less and is further diminished as a function of the duration of incubation. An increase in binding at lower temperature is also seen in the liver membrane system [281]. When I^{125}-insulin binding to circulating cells is studied at 15C° under steady state conditions and B/F of labeled insulin is plotted as a function of the insulin bound (Scatchard plot), two orders of binding sites are apparent, in the circulating lymphocyte cells, isolated from healthy subjects and NIDDM patients before and after long term administration of 1.0 gm oleuropein daily for 6 month..(figure 3-17 a, b, c) the affinity constant of high and low order sites are 2×10^9 and 1.4×10^9, 1.9×10^9 and 1.3×10^9 M^{-1} in healthy subjects and NIDDM patients respectively.

There was no significant difference in the values of the affinity constant in NIDDM patients against the healthy subjects although there is a significant reduce in number of binding sites of each order 1& 2., as shown in table (3-61). A significant effect of diabetic disease was observed on the number of receptors in lymphocyte cell. The affinity constant was not affected although the binding percent was low due to a defect in number of binding sites. From table (3-61) we obtained a significant decrease in binding sites of both orders of sites 210 for order 1 sites and 1200 for order 2 sites compared with 350 binding sites of order 1 and 1700 of order 2 in healthy subjects. While in NIDDM patients who intake 1.0 gm daily of oleuropein for long period of treatment (6 month) the number of binding sites increased to 320 for order sites 1 and 1600 for order sites 2.

Table 3-61. Affinity constants and maximum binding capacity of insulin binding to circulating lymphocytes isolated from healthy subjects, NIDDM patients before and after treatment with 1.0 gm oleuropein daily for 6 months respectively.

Type of group	Type of Binding sites order	Apparent affinity Constant M^{-1}	Number of binding sites
Healthy subjects	1	2.11×0^{9}	350
	2	1.44×10^{9}	1700
NIDDM before OLE intake	1	1.90×10^{9}	210
	2	1.31×10^{9}	1200
NIDDM after OLE intake	1	1.95×10^{9}	320
	2	1.37×10^{9}	1600

The role of insulin in the metabolism of the lymphocyte cells is clear, a number of insulin effects have been demonstrated. Hadden et al reported that insulin stimulates membrane ATPase activity in cultured lymphocytes [282]. Goldfine et al. have demonstrated correlations between the binding of labeled insulin and the ability of insulin to stimulate aminoisobutyric acid uptake in isolated thymic lymphocytes from rats [283], similarly Boyett et al [284] have recently demonstrated the stimulation of glucose transport into thymic lymphocyte by insulin. These studies suggest that it is entirely possible that insulin receptor is employed to biologically significant event. [279]. While the lymphocyte is undoubtedly not a major metabolic target tissue for insulin several lines of evidence suggest that the readily accessible lymphocyte may reflect the physiologic and possibly the pathologic states of the insulin receptor in the major sites of insulin action in liver and fat tissue.

Acher et al, and Cuatrecasas P et al, demonstrated an alteration in the interaction of insulin with receptors on lymphocytes from insulin resistant obese glucose- intolerant patients when compared to thin normal subjects [285-286], these indirect studies further suggest the lymphocyte insulin receptor may be used to reflect events occurring in the major target tissues of insulin action. The similarities between insulin receptors in a human lymphocyte and those in liver and fat cells of rats are striking. Binding of hormone is rapid and reversible process in all three systems. The affinity constants observed in peripheral lymphocytes was consistent with a heterogeneous population of binding sites and are of the same order of magnitude as have been reported in fat cell and liver membrane preparations.

Scatchard analysis suggests that the receptor population of both lymphocyte cells isolated from healthy and NlDDM patients is heterogeneous with respect to equilibrium constant. A similar result has been obtained by Gillman et al [281].

The results may be represented by two orders of sites a high affinity-low capacity and a low affinity-high capacity sites. The difference in observed binding appears to be due to decrease in the number of receptor sites in NIDDM patients. The data presented in series of studies suggest that in this syndrome there is an impairment of the insulin receptors interaction in lymphocyte cell due to a decrease in the number of receptors, especially those of higher affinity. The result is at any insulin concentration the amount of insulin bound by the membranes of the hyperglycemic patients is significantly less than that bound by their normoglycemic subjects.

The value of Ka 1.3×10^9 M^{-1} is typical of the association rate constants for most protein- protein interaction and is similar to several previous studies estimates for insulin binding in other systems employing assumptions concerning binding site number,[287]equilibrium constant [288]. The intrinsic binding constant K_{aff} 2.1×10^9 M^{-1} is in good agreement with that determined graphically for the high affinity component of the scatchard plot slope in Figure (3-17a, b, and c).

Oleuropein may be act by decreasing insulin resistance at the level of muscle and fat, so that the body owns insulin becomes more efficient in its action to control blood glucose, thus OLE may act by binding to sulphonylurea receptors resulting in closure of the membrane K-ATP channels, depolarization of membrane opening of voltage-dependent calcium channels and elevation of intracellular Ca^{++} ions. Possible actions of OLE may include enhancement of β-cell glucose metabolism or activation of enzyme systems generating cyclic AMP or phospholipid derived messengers, in conclusion, the antihyperglycemic action of OLE is associated with the stimulation of insulin secretion and enhancement. Our Preliminary studies in page (132) to evaluate the possible mechanism of fat cell glucose uptake possibly reflect the effect of an active constituent in olive leaves extract. OLE therefore represents an active antihyperglycemic dietary adjunct for the treatment of DM and potential source for discovery of new orally active agents for future diabetic therapy.

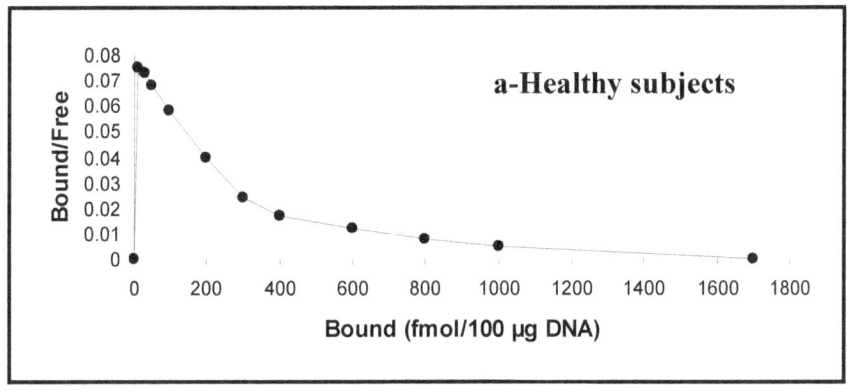

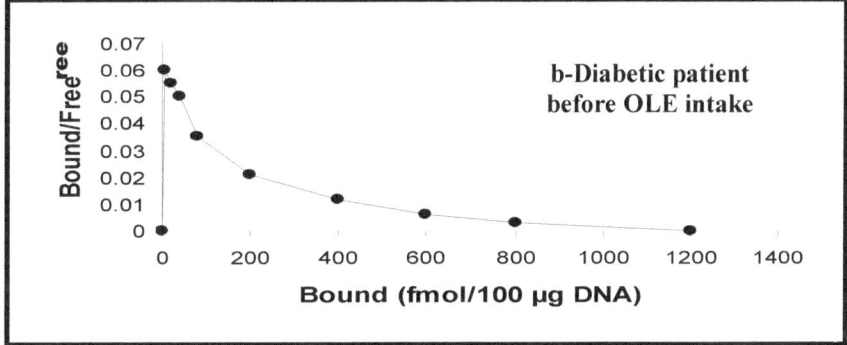

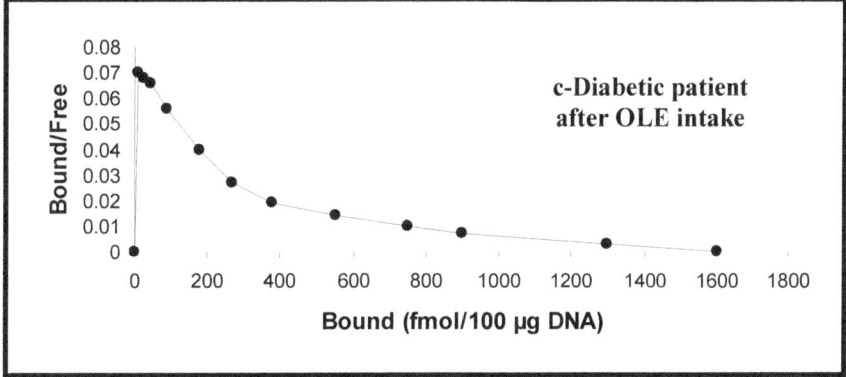

Figure 3-17 a, **b**, and **c**. Plot of Bound/free I^{125}-insulin as a function of insulin bound to lymphocyte cells. Peripheral lymphocytes (1×10^8 cell/ml) were incubated with 1×10^{-11} M I^{125}-insulin.Determination of high order site was made using hormone concentration in the range of 1×10^{-11} to 3×10^{-10}M labeled insulin while data in the range $2 \times 10^{-9} - 2 \times 10^{-7}$ M insulin were analyzed in determination of the low order site. Each point is average of three experiments. All data were corrected for "non-specific-binding" which was about 5 %.

3.9. Histological studies

3.9.1. Histological changes in islets of Langerhans

A- Control islets

Animals of the control group did not appear to have any histological changes during the stages of experiment, since all the islets of the control animals appeared regular in shape with no marked differences between them, small islets of about (21μ) in diameter and reached (38 μ) in large islets. Islets of control animals had well defined boundaries. Most of the cells were of the β-type. β-cells were small polygonal arranged in groups & cords fine capillaries (Fig 3-18).

B-Diabetic islets

First week

The islets of diabetic mice showed variation in size and shape of cells, they also showed moderate beta cell degranulation. Some islets had uneven borders (Fig 3-19, 20). The islets of animals treated with both alloxan and oleuropein appeared to be normal as the control islets with less degranulation and showed activity with the congested blood vessels (Fig 3-21).

The pancreatic of alloxan induced diabetic animals group showed β-cell degranulation which occurs as a rapid event following alloxan intake. These results agree well with that reported by Arison [289]. β-cell degranulation is caused mostly by the deposition of glycogen. The presence of glycogen seems to be related to the duration period of hyperglycemia [290].

On the other hand islets of the alloxan induced diabetic animals treated daily pure oleuropein shows regular shape with less degranulation which means that not all islets or all β-cells are affected at the same rate, since small area of the islet shows almost normal picture. Eventually, islets of hyperglycemia mice are significantly altered with their overall size gradually increasing with the duration and severity of the persistent hyperglycemia.

Second week

In alloxan induced diabetic animals, islets appeared regular in shape, some with hypertrophied cells and large nuclei, this hypertrophy continued and nuclei of cells appeared light. They also showed hyperplasia and early fibrosis. Some islets appear atrophied and show exocrine-endocrine transformation with small thickening of the connective tissue (Fig 3-22, 23, 24). The treated alloxan induced diabetic animals with oleuropein showed islets with regular shape similar to those of control animals with decreased granulation. Almost all cells are completely degranulated. Islets are of normal shape with very few congested blood vessels.

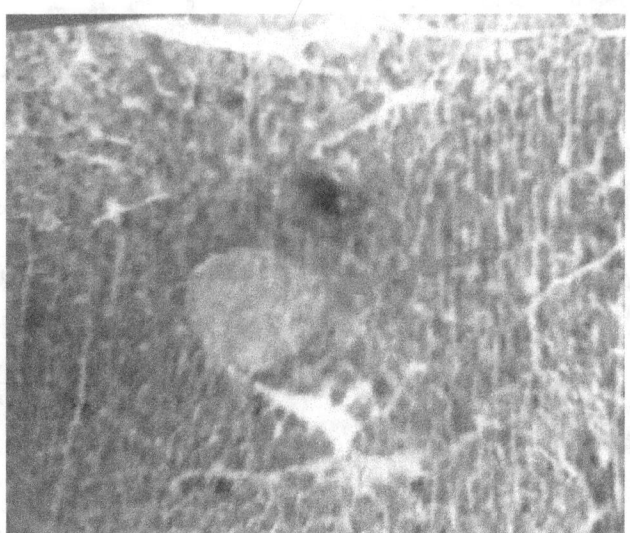

Figure 3-18. Section in a pancreas of the control mice shows a normal islet, regular in shape and size. (330X)

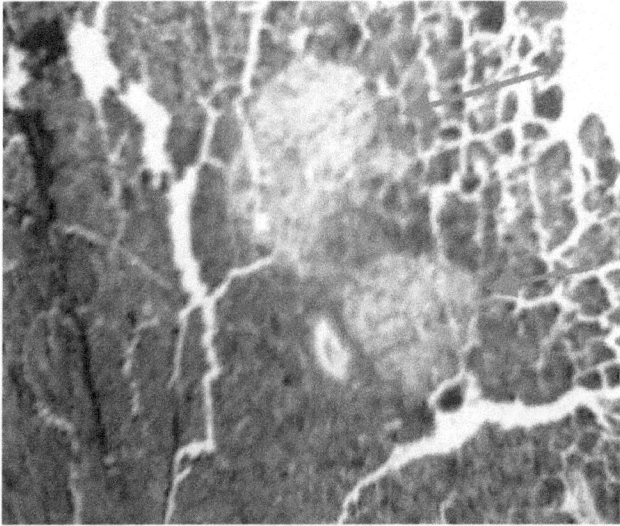

Figure 3-19. Islet of Langerhans of alloxan induced diabetic mice after week of the experiment (330X).

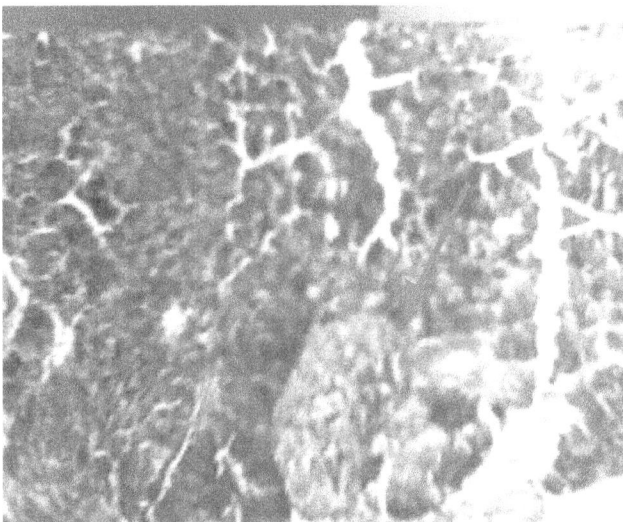

Figure 3-20. Islets of Langerhans of the alloxan induced diabetic mice after one week of the experiment, showing variation in shape and size of the cells with β-cell degranulation (330X)

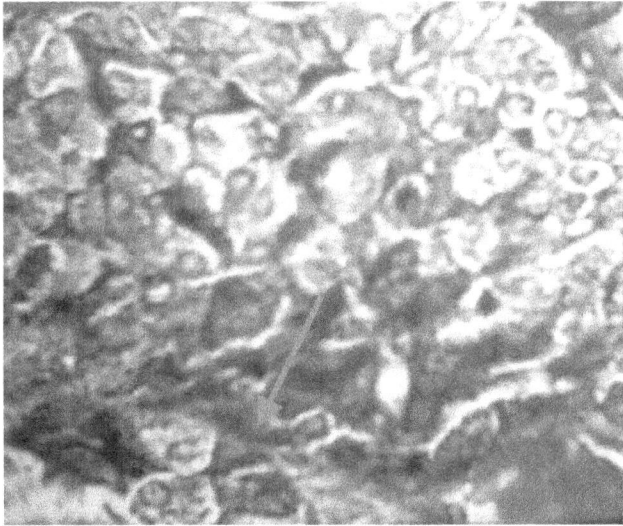

Figure 3-21. A section in the pancreas of the alloxan induced diabetic mice treated with oleuropein on the first week of experiment, shows two islets of Langerhans appear normal like showing activity with the congested blood vessels in the pancreas (1320X)

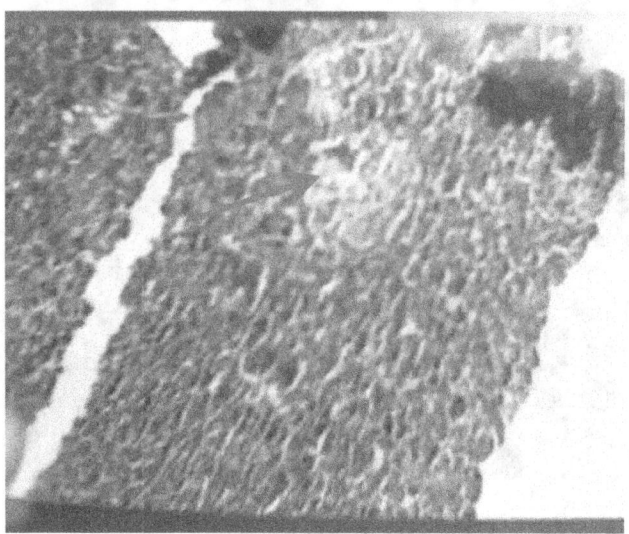

Figure 3-22. Islets of alloxan induced diabetic mice after two weeks of the experiment appear regular in shape with hyperplasia and early fibrosis (330X)

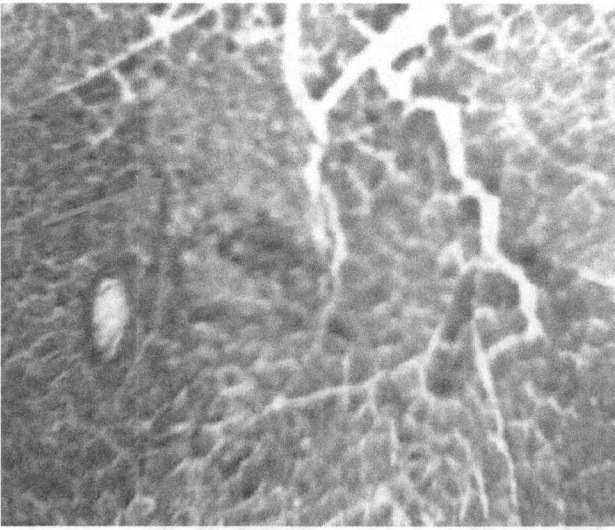

Figure 3-23. Islet of alloxan induced diabetic mice after two weeks of the experiment, showing hyperplasia with large and light nuclei (330 X).

At the second week, islets of alloxan induced diabetic animals show hypertrophy with hyperplasia and this hypertrophy continued to the last week, those islets appeared regular in shape with hypertrophied cells and light nuclei compared with healthy animals group, in addition to the connective tissue was not seen in all the islets as a result of hypertrophy. Some islets appeared atrophoid with dense nuclei.

Third week

At the end of study, the alloxan induced diabetic animals showed continuity of hypertrophy in islets and hyperplasia, associated with infiltration of some of the islets by small lymphocytes (insulitis) with scanty cytoplasm; these infiltrated islets are even larger than normal, since infiltration of mononuclear lymphocyte occurs. In addition to some signs of sclerosis appeared in most of the islet arterioles and this leads to complete occlusion in arterioles due to wall thickening of the arterioles and hyalinization of the intima [291]. Some islets showed lipid accumulation but those islets were rarely seen (Fig 3-25, 26).

The islets of alloxan induced diabetic animals continuously treated with oleuropein showed irregularity in size, but they appeared normal with decreased granulation and some islets appeared atrophoid and very small with few cells. Some of those islets showed few hyperplasias with large dilated blood vessels (Fig 3-27).

Along with the histological studies, the statistical study showed significant results at $p < 0.05$. After the first week of experiment, the alloxan diabetic showed a significant increase in the average of islet diameter, since it was (31 ± 6.5) μ in control group and reached (44.5 ± 9.0) μ in alloxan induced diabetic animals, also there was a significant increase in the experimentally treated by 100 mg/ kg alloxan and oleuropein, so it reached (44.5 ± 6.5) µ compared with control animals (31 ± 6.5) µ..

On the second week of experiment, none of the groups shows any significance at p <0.05. After third week there was significance in diameter of islets between the alloxan induced diabetic animals and the alloxan induced diabetic animals treated daily with pure oleuropein, since it reached (47.3 ± 12.3) µ in alloxan induced diabetic animals compared with (37.2 ± 5.5) µ in treated animals with pure oleuropein .

Table 3-62. The average of islet diameter in µ (Mean ± SD) in both healthy and alloxan induced diabetic mice pre and post treatment with oleuropein.

Animal group	n	Average of islet diameter (µm)		
		1st week	2nd week	3rd week
Healthy mice	6	31 ± 6.5	37.5 ± 6.4	36.5 ± 6.8
Alloxan induced diabetic mice	6	44.5± 9.0	44.3 ± 8.5	47.3 ± 12.3
Alloxan induced diabetic mice treated daily with oleuropein	6	44.5 ± 6.5	42.5 ± 6.4	37.2 ± 5.5

At the last week, alloxan induced diabetic animals showed continuous hypertrophy and hyperplasia in islets in addition to sclerosis and insulitis. It is worthily to mention that the increase in islet diameter and number were shown as hypertrophy and hyperplasia, this was significantly shown as an increase in alloxan induced diabetic animals at the last week compared with healthy group.

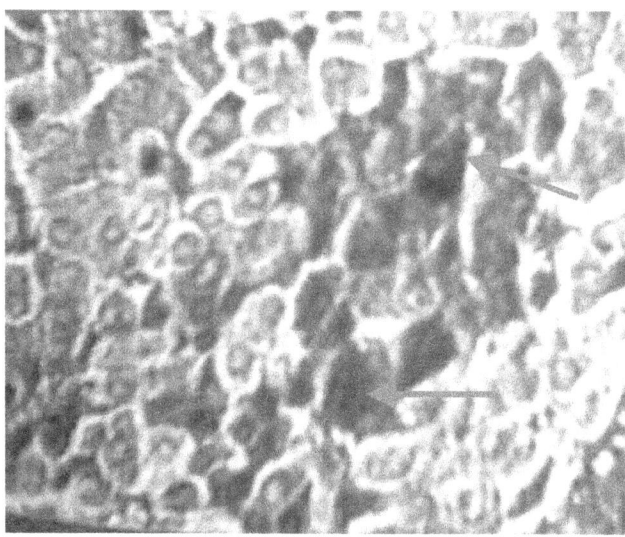

Figure 3-24. Islet of alloxan induced diabetic mice after two weeks of the experiment, shows hypertrophy with exocrine-endocrine transformation (1320 X)

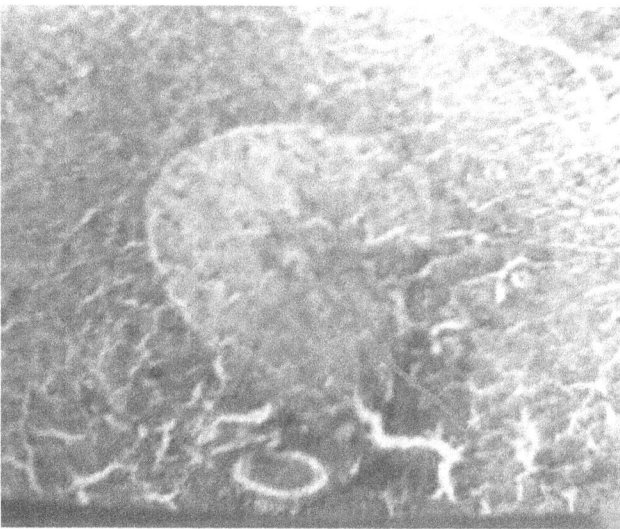

Figure 3-25. Islet of alloxan induced diabetic mice after three weeks of the experiment, shows hypertrophy and hyperplasia with infiltration by lymphocytes (insulitis) (330 X)

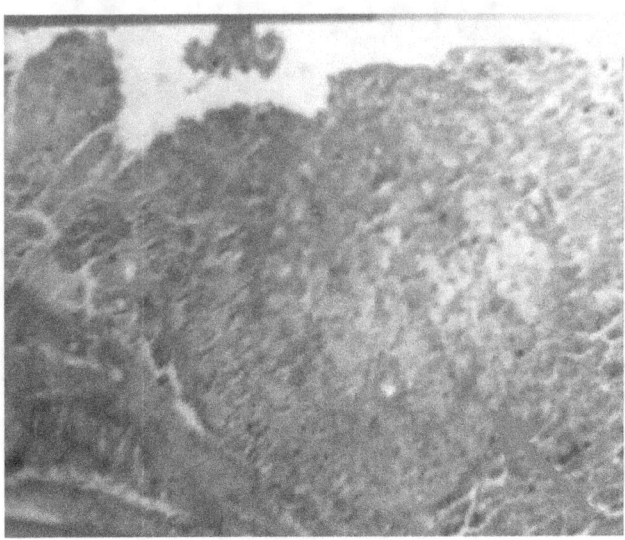

Figure 3-26. Islet of alloxan induced diabetic mice after three weeks of the experiment, shows hypertrophy with scanty cytoplasm of the β-cells. (330 X)

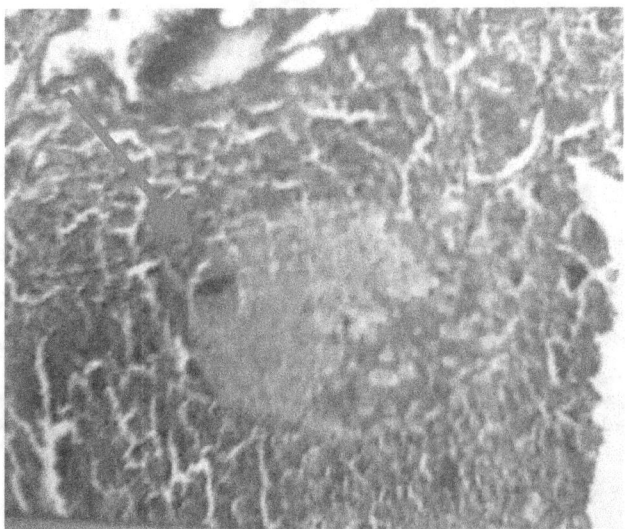

Figure 3-27. Two islets of Langerhans of alloxan induced diabetic mice treated with oleuropein for three weeks appear normal with few atrophoid cells (330X)

Insulitis is associated mostly with lymphocyte infiltration which has been noticed in chronic juvenile diabetes similar to those of Freyse [292] , this increase in lymphocyte cells has been produced by a simple immune response which causes necrosis of islets or anti insulin serum injection, also small doses of the toxin (alloxan or streptozotocin) as reported by Volk[293], those two authors also reported a hyalinization of the media causes thickening in the wall of the arterioles which leads in some cases to partial or complete occlusion of the arterioles, similar to results found by Freyse and Volk. [292,293]

Islets of the alloxan induced diabetic animals treated daily with pure oleuropein showed irregularity in size, with few small islets which were atrophied as a result of their activity. Most of the islets showed hyperplasia but all of the islets appeared normal as of the healthy group.

Previous experimental studies that have used different traditional plant extracts such as (Artemisia herbal Alba, blueberry, juniper berries. etc.) have investigated the effect of those plants on blood glucose and insulin levels. However, they did not elucidate the effect of those plant extracts on the pancreatic islets [294,295].

Finally the present study has illustrated for the first time the effect of secoiridoid phenolic compound isolated from olive leaves (oleuropein) on the pancreatic islets and discussed those changes with the levels of blood glucose and oxidative stress status in alloxan induced diabetic animals.

CONCLUSIONS

1) Oleuropein considered as hypoglycemic agent reduce oxidative stress, indirectly by lowering blood glucose and preventing hyperinsulinemia and directly by acting as free radical scavengers.

2) Oleuropein supplementation is associated with a protective effect against coronary heart disease. Specifically oleuropein administration of as little as 500 mg daily can make LDL less susceptible to oxidation and consequently less atherogenic.

3) Oleuropein is generally safe and effective in reducing symptoms of diabetic peripheral neuropathy.

4) Oleuropein reduced lipid peroxidation in diabetic patients, improvement the total antioxidant capacity, reduced LDL-cholesterol, reduced uric acid.

5) Oleuropein considered a broad natural antibiotic effective in killing most microorganisms.

6) Oleuropein have a significant effect on increasing number of receptors and improvement insulin action

7) Oleuropein supplementations significantly improve glycemic control possibly by minimizing free radical damage to the pancreatic β-cells.

8) Oleuropein have a direct protective effect on β-cells against alloxan damaging the islets of Langerhans.

References

1) Privitera JR, *Olive Leaf Extract*: A New/Old Healing Bonanza for Mankind Covina, CA: NutriScreen, Inc., 1996.

2) Panizzi LM, Scarpati JM, Oriente EG. *Gazzetta Chimica Italiana* (1960); 90: 1449–1485.

3) Esdorn I. *Planta Med* (1954) 2:145

4) Stegmann K.*Landartz* (1954) 15:375.

5) Riberiro Rde A, Fiuza deMelo MM, De Barros F. *J Ethnopharmacol* (1986); 15: 261.

6) Circosta C, Occhiuto A, Gregorio S. *Planta Med Phytother.* (1960); 24:264.

7) Zarzuelo A, Duarte J, Jimenez J. *Planta Med* (1991); 57: 417.

8) Visioli F and Galli C. *Life Sci* (1994); 55: 1965–1971.

9) Petkov V and Manolov P. *Drug Res* (1972); 22: 1476.

10) Peirce A. *Practical Guide to Natural Medicines*. New York: William Morrow and Co. (1999): 469-71.

11) Visoli F and Galli C. *Nutr Rev* (1998); 56:142-147.

12) Coni E, Benedetto M, Pasquale R, Masella D, Modesti R, Mattei and EA. *Lipids* (2000); 35(1):45-54.

13) Visoli F, and Galli C. *Atheroscler* Rep. (2000); 3: 64-67.

14) Mohamed T, Khayyal M, Mona A, El-Ghazaly D, Abdalaha N, Nassar N, Okpanyi, and Matthias H. *Drug Res.* (2002); 52:797-802.

15) Wern RC. Potterss New Cyclopedia of Botanical Drugs and Preperation Essex, England: CW DanialCo. (1985): 204.

16) Walker M, "*Natures Antibiotic olive Leaf Extract*" Kensington Publishing Corp. New York, (1997).

17) Pooley RJ and Peterson LR. "Mechanisms of microbial susceptibility and resistance to antimicrobial agents." *In* The Biologic and Clinical Basis of Infectious Diseases, 5th Edition. Editors ST, Shulman JP, Phair LR, Peterson JR. (Philadelphia: W.B. Saunders Company), p. 550, (1997).

18) Renis HE. Antimicrobial *Agents and Chemotherapy* (1970); 3: 167-168.

19) Elliot GA, Buthala DA, DeYoung EN. *Antimicrobial Agents and Chemotherapy* (1969); 3:173-176.

20) Tassou CC, Nychas GJ, Board, RG. *Biotechnology Applied Biochemistry* (1991); 13: 231-237.

21) Somova L, Shode FO, and Ramnanan P. *J Ethinopharmacol* (2003); 84:299-305.

22) Diaz A, Abad M, Fernandez L. *Biol Pharm Bull* (2000); 23: 1307-1313.

23) Ghisalberti E. *Phytomedicine* (1998); 5: 147-163.

24) Visoli F and Galli C. *Atherosclerosis* (1995); 117:25-32.

25) Tuck KL and Hayball PJ. *Nutr Biochem* (2002); 11:636-644.

26) Onderoglu S, Sozer KM, Erbil R and Lermioglu F. *J Pharm Pharmacol* (1999); 51(11):1305-1312.

27) Gonzalez M, Zarzuelo, MJ, Gamez MP, Utrilla J Jimenez and IOsuna. *Planta Med* (1992); 8(6): 513-515.

28) Pinelli P, Romani A, Vincieri F, Mullinacci N. *J Agric Food Chem* (1999); 47:964-967.

29) Benavent O, Castillo J, LKorente. *J Food Chem* (2000); 68:457- 462.

30) Le Toutour B, Guedon D. *Phytochemistry* (1992); 31:1173–1178.

31) Fredkinson WR, U.S. Patant 6117844; Appl.No.668324; September 12, (2000).

32) *Olive leaf Extract-Natures Antibiotic*, Dr. Morton. Kensington Publishing Corp. (1997).

33) Konlee M, *The olive leaf.* Positive Health News, No 11, spring (1996) (Keep Hope Alive, PO Box 27041, West Allis, WI, 53227).

34) Benkhalti F, Legssyer A, Gomez P, Perez-Jimenez F and Boustani ES.*Therapie* (2003); 2:133-137.

35) De la Puerta R, Ruiz-Gutierrez V, Hoult JR. *Biochem Pharmacol* (1999); 57:445–449.

36) Perricone Nicholas V. W.O. Patant WO1076579; APPL.No. 20000623. October 18, (2001).

37) Fleming HP, Walter WM, Tchells JL. *Microbiology* (1973); 26:777-782.

38) Bourquelot E, Vintilesco J. *CR Acad Sci* (1908); 147:533–535.

39) Ruiz-Guterrez, Martin-Domingues and de la Puerta. *J Agric food Chem* (2000); 55:814-819.

40) Loweenstein CJ, Hill SH, Walker AL, Wu J. *J Clin Invest* (1996); 97:1837-1834.

41) Boskou D. *Wld Rev Nutr Diet* (2000); 87: 56–77.

42) Brenes M, Garcia A, Garcia J, and Garrido J. *J Agric Food Chem* (1999); 47: 3535.

43) Amoit JM and Fleuriet. *JAgric Food Chem* (1989); 28:67.

44) Amiot MJ, Fleuriet A, Macheix JJ. *J Agric Food Chem* (1986); 34:823–826.

45) Montedoro G, Servili M, Baldioli M and Miniati E. *J Agric Food Chem* (1993) ; 41:2228-2234.

46) Montedoro G, Servili M, Baldioli M and Miniati E. *J Agric Food Chem* (1992); 40:1571–1576.

47) Limiroli R, Cossonni R, Ranalli A, and Zetta L. *J Chem Soc Perkin Trans.*(1) (1995) ; 44:1519-1523. .

48) Cimato A, Modi G, Alessandri S, Mattei A. *'informatore Agrario* (1992); 18:55–75.

49) Steinberg D, Parthasarathy S, Carew TE, Khoo JC, Witzum JL. *New Engl J Med* (1989); 320: 915–924.

50) Visioli F and Galli C. *J Agric Food Chem* (1998); 46:4292-4296.

51) Visioli F and Galli C. *Nutr Metab Cardiovasc Dis.* (1997); 7: 459–466.

52) Aruoma OI, Deiana M, Jenner A, Halliwell B, Harparkash K, Banni S . *J Agric Food Chem.* (1998); 46: 5181–5187.

53) Visoli F, Bellomo G, and Galli C. *Biochem Biophy Res Coummun* (1998); 247:60-65.

54) Aruoma OI, Halliwell B. *Biochem J* (1987); 248: 973–976.

55) Rice-Evans CA, Miller NJ, Paganga G. *Free Rad Biol Med* (1996); 20: 933–956.

56) Dieana M, Aruoma OI, Bianchi ML, Spoencer JP. *Free Rad Biol Med.* (1999); 26: 762- 769.

57) Petroni A, Blasevich M, Salami M, Papini N, Montedoro GF, Galli C. *Thromb Res.* (1995); 78: 151–160.

58) Kohyama N, Nagata T, Fujimoto S, Sekiya K. *Biosci Biotech Biochem.* (1997); 61: 347–350.

59) Visioli F, Petroni A, Galli C. Phenolic compounds extracted from olive oil prevents oxidation of low density lipoproteins, and inhibit platelet function and platelet and leukocyte eicosanoid production in vitro. *In*: Paoletti R, Samuelsson B, Catapano AL, Poli A, Rinetti M, editors. Oxidative processes and antioxidants. New York: Raven Press; (1994) pp 199–206.

60) Scaccini C, Nardini M, D'Aquino M, Gentili V, Di Felice M, Tomassi G. *J Lipid Res* (1992); 33: 627–633.

61) Wiseman SA, Mathot JN, de Fouw NJ, Tijburg LB. *Atherosclerosis.* (1996); 120: 15–23.

62) Bonanome A, Pagnan A, Caruso D, Toia A, Xamin AF. *Nutr Metab Cardiovasc Res (*2000); 12: 450-460.

63) Bourne LC, Rice-Evans CA. *Free Rad Res* (1998); 28: 429–438.

64) Bravo L. *Nutr Rev.* (1999); 56: 317–333.

65) Visioli F, Galli C, Bornet F, Mattei A, Patelli R, Galli G. *FEBS Lett* (2000) 468:159–160.

66) Manna C, Galletti P, Cucciolla V, Montedoro G, Zappia V. *J Nutr Biochem* (1999); 10: 159–165.

67) Bliekas G, Vassilkis C, Tisimidou, M, and Boskou D. *J Agric Food Chem* (2002); 50: 3688-3692.

68) Boskou D.*World Rev.Nutr.Diet.* (2000); 87: 56-77.

69) Stark AH and Msadar Z. *Nutr Rev* (2002); 60: 170-176.

70) Vissers MN, Zock PL, Leenen R and Katan, M B. *J Nutr.* (2002); 132: 409-417.

71) Micro-Cases E, Govas, M and De la Torre, R. *Eur J Clin Nutr.* (2003); 57: 186-190.

72) Bai C, Yan X, Nagata. *J Agric Food Chem.* (1998); 46: 3998.

73) Wiseman, SA, Tijburg LB, and van de Put, F H. *Lipids.* (2002); 37: 1053-1057.

74) Angelo S, Manna C, Migliardi V, Capossi G. *Drug Metab Dispos* (2001) 29: 1492-1498.

75) Piero Del B, Antonietta D, Amalia D, Nicolla C, and Licia I . *J Chromatography* (2003); 785:47-56.

76) Augustein S and Gray W. *J Nut.* (2000); 130: 2073S-2085S.

77) Azar M, Verette E, Brun S. *J Food Sci.* (1987); 52: 1255–1257.

78) Fernández de Simón B, Pérez-Ilzarbe J, Hernández T, Gómez-Cordovés C, Esterella I. *Chromatogr* (1990); 30: 35–37.

79) Fernández de Simón B, Pérez-Ilzarbe J, Hernández T, Gómez-Cordovés C, Estrella I. *J Agric Food Chem* (1992); 40: 1531–1535.

80) Tomás-Lorente F, García-Viguera C, Ferreres F, Tomás-Barberán FA. *J Agric Food Chem* (1992); 40: 1800–1804.

81) Kanes K, Tisserat B, Berhow M, Vandercook C. *Phytochem* (1993); 32: 967–974.

82) Goupy PM, Varoquaux PJA, Nic Ola JJ, Macheix JJ. *J Agric Food Chem* (1990); 38: 2116–2121.

83) Lee HS, Widmer BW. *Phenolic compounds.* In: Nollet LML, ed. Handbook of Food Analysis. Physical Characterization and Nutriet Analysis. New York, USA: Marcel Dekker, Inc., (1996); Vol 1, p.821–894.

84) Kuninori T, Nishiyama J. *J Chromatogr* (1986); 362: 255–262.

85) Rommel A, Wrolstad RE. *J Agric Food Chem* (1993a); 41: 1237–1241.

86) Robards K, Prenzler PD, Tucker G, Swatsitang P, Glover W. *Food Chem* (1999); 66: 401–436.

87) Nishibe S and Sugawara A.*Natural Medicines* (2002) ;1:18-22

88) Finger A, Engelhardt UH, Wray V. *J Sci Food Agric* (1991); 55: 313–321.

89) MoulyP, Gaydou EM, Estienne J. *J Chromatogr* (1993) 634: 129–134.

90) Schmidt TJ, Merfort I, Willuhn G. *J Chromatogr* A (1994);'69: 236–240.

91) Angerosa F, d'Alessandro N, Konstantinou P. & Di Giacinto L. *J Agric Food Chem*(1995); 43: 1802

92) Vande Casteele K, Geiger H, van Sumere CF. *J Chromatogr* (1983); 258: 111–124. S

93) Lamuela-Raventós RM, Waterhouse AL. *Am J Enol Vitic* (1994); 45: 1–5.

94) Marko-Varga G, Barcelo D. *Chromatogr* (1992); 34: 146–154.

95) Merken HM, Beecher GR.: A review. *J Agric Food Chem* (2000); 48: 577–599.

96) Delage E, Baron GB, Drilleau J-F. *J Chromatogr* (1991); 555: 125–136.

140) Uzel N, Sivas A, Uysal M, Oz H. *Horm Metab Res* (1987); 19:89–90.

141) Cser A, Sziklai LI, Menzel H, Lombeck I. *Trace Elem Electroly* (1993); 7: 205–10.

142) Asayama K, Hayashibe H, Dobashi K, Níitsu T, Miyao A, Kato K. *Diabetes Res* (1989); 12: 85–91.

143) Szaleczky E, Prechl J, Pusztai P, Rosta A, Fehér J, Somogyi A. *Med Sci Monit* (1997); 3:163–6.

144) Prechl J, Szaleczky E, Pusztai P, Kocsis I, Tulassay Zs, Somogyi A. *Med Sci Monit* (1997); 3: 167–70.

145) Wolf SP, Dean RT. *Biochem J* (1987); 245:243–50.

146) Williamson JR, Chang K, Frangos M. *Diabetes* (1993); 42: 801–13.

147) Nito M. *N Engl J Med* (1993); 32: 977–86.

148) Pieper GM, Langenstroer P, Gross GJ. *Mol Cell Biochem* (1993); 122: 139–45.

149) Cao G, Booth SL, Sadowski JA, and Prior RL. *Am J Clin Nutr* (1998); 68:1081–1087.

150) Steinberg D. *Lancet* (1995); 346:36-38.

151) Salonen JT, Nyyssonen K, Tuomainen T-P, Maenpaa PH, Korpela H, Kaplan GA, Lynch LJ, and Helmrich SP, Salonen R. *Br J Med* (1999); 311: 1124–1127.

152) Ihara Y, Toyokuni S, Uchida K, Odaka H, Tanaka T, Ikeda H, Hiai H, Seino Y, and Yamada Y. *Diabetes* (1999); 48:927–932.

153) Rimm EB, Stampfer MJ, Ascherio A, Giovanniucci E, Colditz GA, Willet WC. *N Eng J Med* (1993); 328:1450–1456.

154) Kubota A, Hiai H, and Seino Y. *FEBS Lett* (2000); 73:24–26.

155) Sen CK, Roy S, and Packer L: Alpha-lipoic acid: cell regulatory function and potential therapeutic implications. In Packer L, Hiramatsu M, Yoshikawa T (Eds): "Antioxidant Food Supplements in Human Health." New York: Academic (1999). pp 111–119.

156) Ziegler D, Hanefeld M, Ruhnau KJ, Meissner HP, Lobisch M, Schutte K, Gries F. *Diabetol* (1995); 38: 1425–1433.

157) Ziegler D, Gries FA. *Diabetes* (1997); 36 (Suppl 2):62S–66S.

158) Ziegler D, Hanefeld M, Ruhnau KJ, Hasche H, Lobisch M, Schutte K, and Kerum G, Malessa R. *Diabetes* (1999); 22: 1296–1301.

159) Lean ME, Noroozu M, Kelly I, Burns J, and Talwar D, Sattar Crozier A. *Diabetes* (1999); 48:176–181.

160) Ford ES, Will JC, Bowman BA, and Narayan KM. *Am J Epidem* (1999); 149:168.

161) Trachtman H, Futterweit S, Maneska J, Ma C, Valderrama Fuchs A, Tarectecan AA, Rao PS, Sturman JA, Boles TH, Fu Baynes J . *Am J Physiol* (1995); 269: F429–F438.

162) Singh RB, Niaz MA, Rastogi SS, Shukla PK, Thakur AS. *J Hypertens* (1999); 13: 203–208

163) Nachman, Leslie (USA). *Patant* No. 5714150, Appl. No.780448, Feb (1998).

164) Singleton VL and Rossi JA. *Am J Enol Vitic* (1965); 16: 144-158.

165) Cyril S, Raid E, and Frida D. *J Agric Food Chem* (2002); 49:618-621.

166) Servili M, Baldioli M, Selvaggini R, Macchioni A, & Montedoro G. *J Agric Food Chem* (1999); 47:12.

167) Brene M, Garcia J, Rios A.. *J Agric Food Chem* (1999); 47: 3530.

168) Gariboldi G, Jommi G and Verotta I. *Phytochemistry* (1986); 25:865-870.

169) Cyril S, Beatrice, Riad E, Frida D, Kamel B and Guy B. *J Agric Food Chem* (2001); 49: 618-621.

170) Limiroli R, Consonni R, and lina G. *J Chem Soc Perkin Trans.* (1995); 1: 1519-1523.

171) Balla G, Jacob H, Eaton J, Belcher J. Hemin. *Arterioscler Thromb* (1991); 11: 1700-1711.

172) Visoli F, Petroni A and GalliC. *Fatty acids.* (1997b); 57:212.

173) Zhen-Dan He, Paul Pui-Hay But, Tak-Wah Doominic Chan and Han-Dong Sun. Chem *Pharm Bull* (2001); 49:780-784.

174) Re R, Pellegrini N, Proteggente A, Pannala A, Yang M, Rice-Evans C. y. *Free Rad Biol Med* (1999); 26:1231-1237.

175) David T, Plummer. *An introduction to practical biochemistry* .2ed McGRAW-HILL Book company (UK) Limited.

176) Jansson L and Sandler S. *Pathol Anat* (1986);410:17-21

177) Trinder P. *Ann Clin Biochem* (1969); 6:24-27.

178) Makarem A. Clinical Chemistry-Principles and Twechniques.2nd .R.F.Henery, D.C.Cannon, J.W.Winkelman, Editors. Harper and Row, Hagetsrstown (1974); 1128-1135.

179) Standderfor NY. *Clin Chem* (1987); 32: 1269.

180) Richmond W. *Clin Chem* (1973); 19: 1350-1356.

181) Burstein M. *Lipid Res* (1970); 11: 583.

182) Friedewald WT, Levy RI, and Frederickson DS. *Clin Chem* (1972); 18: 499-502.

183) Fossatti P, Prencipel. *Clin.Chem* (1982); 28: 2077.

184) Artiss JD. Clin Chem Acta (1981); 116:301-309.

185) Chaney AL, Patton CJ, and Crouch SR. *Anal Chem* (1977); 49: 464-469.

186) Husdan H.*Clin.Chem* (1968); 14: 222-238.

187) Peters T. *Clin Chem* (1968); 14: 1147.

188) Doumas BT, Waston WA, Biggs HG. *Clin Chim Acta* (1971); 31:87.

189) Monnet L. *Annal Biol Clin* (1963); 21:717.

190) Frankle S and Reitman S. *Amer J clin Path* (1957); 28: 56.

191) Belefield A, Goldberg DM. *Enzyme* (1971); 12: 561.

192) Ohkawa H, Ohishi Na, and Yagi K. *Anal Biochem* (1979); 95: 351-358.

193) Tietz NW (1984): *Fundamental of Clinical Chemistry* (3rd ed). WB Saunders co.

194) Beutler E. *In* Functions of Glutathione. (Nobel Conf.). Ravan Press. 1969: p.65.

195) Paglia DE, Valentine WN. *J Lab Clin Med* (1967); 30:158.

196) Pleban PA, Muny AB. *Clin Chem* (1982); 28: 311-316.

197) West M, Berger C, Rony H. *J Clin Lab Med* (1961); 57: 946.

198) Lee KT, Tan IK, Seet AM. *Clin Chem Acta* (1975); 58:101-105.

199) Aebihuge A. *Methods in Enzymatic Analysis*. (1974): Vol 2:674-684.

200) Benzie F, Chung WY, and Tomlinson B. *Clinical Chemistry* (1999); 45: 901-904.

201) Bieri JC, Tolliver TJ, Catignari GL. *Am J Clin Nutr* (1979); 32: 2143-2149.

202) Lin. P. *Clin Chem* (1982); 28: 2225-2228.

203) Bieri JC, Brown ED, Smith JC. *J Liquid Chrom* (1995); 8: 473-484.

204) Rice –Evan, NJ and Miller. *Methods Enzymol* (1994); 234:279.

205) Bauer AW, Kirby JC and Turck M. *Am J Clin Pathol* (1966); 45:493-496.

206) Ericsson HM and Sherris JC. *Acta Pathol Microbiol Scand.*(1971);217:1-9

207) World Health Organization Technical Report Service.1977.RepNo.610, WHO Genova.

208) Al-Azzawie. H.F. (1986). M.Sc.Thesis, Univ. of Baghdad.

209) Gaven JR, Gorden P, Archer J. *J Biol Chem* (1975); 248:2202-2208.

210) Burton OH, Rosebrough NW, Farr AL and Randall RJ. *Biochem J.* (1956); 62: 315-317.

211) Cignarella A, Nastasi M, Cavalli E, Puglisi L. *Thrombosis Res* (1996) 84:311-322.

212) Bancroft JD and Steven A. Theory and practice of Histological Techniques 2 Ed .Chjurchill, Livingston. London.

213) Al-Skhaih MN. M.Sc. Thesis, Univ. of Baghdad.

214) Slidders, W. *J Path Bact* (1961) 82:532-543.

215) Rice-Evan CA, Miller NJ Paganga G. *Free Rad Biol Chem* (2000); 21:933-956.

216) Mosca l, De MarcoC, Visoli F, Cannella C. *J Agric Food Chem* (2000); 48:297-301.

217) Ellis R, Vidal O, Diaz L, and Mailrand CI. *J Pharm Belg* (1991); 46:L177-181.

218) Rovellini N, Cortesi E, and Fideli R. *Ital Sostanze Grasse* (1997); 74:273.

219) Ginberg H. *Diabetes* (1996); 45: 27.

220) Schwab U, Malirata M, Sarkkiner S. *Metabolism* (1996); 45:142.

221) Groemer LE, Ramshort EM, Kata MB, and Mensink RP. *Atherosclersis* (1991); 87:239.

222) Koizumi J, Mabuchi H, and Yoshimuri A. *Atherosclersis* (1985); 58:175.

223) Lavie CJ, and McCallister Y. *Clin Proc* (1995); 70: 69.

224) Genest JJ, and Cohn JS. *Am J Cardiol* (1995); 67: 8.

225) Bonanome A, Pagnan A, Caurso D, Toia A. *Nutr Metab Cardiovasc Dis* (1992) ; 10:111.

226) Visoli F, Galli C. *Rev Food Sci Nutr* (2002); 42: 209-221.

227) Bianca F. *J Nutr* (2000); 130:1124-1131.

228) Carmen DJ. *Eur J Clin Invest* (1999); 29: 12-18.

229) Habeeb G. *Belgian Pharmacology Journal* (1994); 49(2:101-108.

230) Lee J, Sparrow D, Vokonas PS, and Landsberg L, Weiss ST. *Am J Epidemiol* (1995); 142:288 –294.

231) Selby JV, Friedman GD, Quesenberry CPJ. *Am J Epidemiol* (1990); 131:1017– 1027.

232) Zavaroni I, Mazza S, Fantuzzi M, Dall'Aglio E, Bonora E, Delsignore R, Passeri M, Reaven GM. *Int J Med* (1993); 234:25–30.

233) Ferris TF, Gorden P. *Am J Med* (1993); 19: 359 –365.

234) Messerli FH, Frohlich ED, Dreslinski GR, Suarez DH, Aristimuno GG. *Ann Intern Med* (1980); 93: 817– 821.

235) Kobrin I, Frohlich ED, Ventura HO, Messerli FH. *Arch Intern Med* (1986); 146:272–276.

236) Cappuccio FP, Strazzullo P, Farinaro E, Trevisan M. *JAMA* (1993); 270:354 – 359.

237) DeFronzo RA, Ferranini E. *Diabetes Care* (1991); 14:173–194.

238) Kooy NW and Royall JA. *Arch Biochem Biophys* (1994); 310: 352–359.

239) Steinberg HO, Brechtel G, Johnson A, Fineberg N, Baron AD. *J Clin Invest* (1994); 94: 1172–1179.

240) Törry JP, Niskanen LK, La¨nsimies EA, Partanen KP, Uusitupa MIJ. *Stroke* (1996); 27: 1316 –1318.

241) Baynes JW. *Diabetes* (1991); 40:405– 412.

242) Becker BF. *Free Radic Biol Med* (1993); 14: 615– 631.

243) Baynes JW. *Diabetes* (1992); 45:407– 412.

244) Suarna C, Dean RT, May J, Stocker R. *Arterioscler Thromb Vasc Biol* (1995); 15: 1616–1624.

245) Fuster V, Badimon L, Badimon JJ, Chesebro JH. *N Engl J Med* (1992); 326: 310 –318.

246) Feingold KR, Grunfeld C. *Diabetes* (1992); 41(suppl 2):97–101.

247) Visy J, Le-Coz P, Chadefaux B, Fressinaud C, Woimant F, Marquet J, Zittoun J,VisyJ,VallatJM,HaquenauM. *Neurology* (1991); 41:1313–1315.

248) Kuwano K, Ikeda H, Oda T, Nakayama H, Koga Y, Toshima H, Imaizumi T. *Am J Physiol* (1996); 270:1993–1999.

249) Sinclair AJ .*Diabetes care*.(1993);2:7-10

250) Oberly LW. *Free Radic Biol Med* (1988); 5:113-124.

251) Griesmacher A, Kiindhauser M, Andert SE, Scvreiner W and Toma C. *Am J Med* (1995); 98: 469-475.

252) Laakksonen DE, Atalay M, Niskanen L, Uiritupa M, Haninen O and Sen CK. *Diabetic care* (1996); 19:569-574.

253) Vaelazquez E, Winocour PH, Kesteven P and Albets KG. *Diabet Med* (1991); 8: 752-758.

254) Bray RC, Cockle SA, Martin E, Roberts PB and Rotillo G. *Biochem J* (1974) ; 139:34-48

255) Ceriello A, Giugliano D, Quatraro A.Dello R, Lefevre PJ. *Diabet Med* (1991); 8:540-542.

256) Michiels C, Raes M, Toussaint O, Remache J. *Free Radic Biol Med* (1994); 17:235-248.

257) Berg EA. *Biochemi* (1995); 77: 919-924.

258) Zhae W. *Free Radic Re*s (1998); 29:315-320.

259) Jain SK and McVie R. *Metabolism* (1994); 43: 306-309.

260) Murakami K, Kondo T, Ohtsuka Y, Fujiwara Y. *Metabolism* (1989); 38:753-758.

261) Ou P, Nourooz-Zadeh J.and Tritscher HJ. *Free Radic Res* (1996); 25:337-3456.

262) Murakami K, Kondo T, Ohtsuka Y, Fujji W and Shimada M. *Metabolism* (1989); 38:753-758.

263) Halliwell B. *Lancet* (1994); 344:72-724.

264) Jos J, Rybak M, Patin PH, Robert JJ, Boitard C and Thevenin R. *Diabetes Metab* (1990); 16: 498.

265) Carmen D. *Diabetes Care* (1998); 21: 1736-1744.

266) Arslanian S, Becker D, Drash A: Diabetes mellitus in the child and adolescent .In The Diagnosis and Treastment of Endocrine Disorder in Childhood and Adolescent.Kappy MS, Blizzard RM, Migeon CJ, EDS.Spring field,II.Thomas 1994,P.961-1026.

267) Frei B, Carr A, Tijerina T, Frei B. *Biochem J* (2000); 346:491–499.

268) Will JC, Byers T. *Nutr Rev* (1996); 54:193-202.

269) Jacob RA. *Diabetes Re*s (1988); 58:312-320.

270) Frei B. *Am J Med* (1994); 97: 5S-13S.

271) Tsuchihashi H, Kigoshi M, Iwatsuki M and Niki E. *Arch.Biochem Biophy* (1995); 323:137-147.

272) Visoli F, Bellomo G, and Galli C. *Biochem Biophys Res Commun* (1998); 247: 60-64.

273) Babich H and Visoli F. *Farmco* (2003); 58(5):403-407.

274) Farag RS, El-Baroty GS, Busuny AM. *J Food Sci Nutr* (2003); 54:159-174.

275) Foggs AH and Lodge, RM.*Trans Faraday Soc.* (1945); 41: 359-364.

276) Juven B, Samish Z. *J appl Bact (1970)*; 33:721.

277) Walter, M. *Townsend letters for Doctors and Patients* 156. July (1993).

278) Kubo I, Matsumoto A, and Takase I. *J Chem Ecol* (1985); 11:251-263.

279) Kono K, Chikara H, and Hiroe Y. *Proc Natl Acad Sci.USA* (1999); 96:9159-9164.

280) Kubo I., Matsumoto A. and Ichiro T. *J.Chem Ecol* (1991) 17:1123-1133.

281) Gilliman JR, Roth J, and Freychet, P. *Proc Nat Acad Sci* (1975); 69:747-751.

282) Hadden JW, Hadden EM and Wilson, E.E. *Proc Nat.Acad Sci.* (1972) 68:1833-1837.

283) Goldfine I, Kahn C, Nevil D and Roth J. *J clin Invest* (1973) ;24:500-510

284) Boyett JD and Hofert JF. *Horm Metab Res.* (1972); 48:135-142.

285) Archer J, Gorden P and Gavin J. *J Clin Metab*(1975);250 :5400-5412

286) Cuatrecasas P, Kahn C, Nevil D and Roth J. *J Biol Chem* (1971); 246:7265-7274.

287) Pierre de Meyts.,Jess R, David M, Nevil J, James R and Gaven L. *J Biol Chem* (1976); 251: 1877-1883.

288) Sherman BM, Gorden, P and Nevil DM. *J Clin Invest* (1971)10; 50:849-858.

289) Arison RN, Ciaccio EI, Glitzer SC, and Pruss MP. *Diabetes(*1967) 16:51-56

290) Lazarus SS and Shapiro SH. *Diabetes* (1972) 21:129-137.

291) Atkins W, and Matty AJ, *J. Endocrinol* (1973) 58:2330-2338.

292) Freyse EJ, Dorsche HH, and Fisher U. *Acta Biol Med Germ* (1982) 41:1203-1210

293) Volk BW and Wellmann KF. Historical Review in: The Diabetic pancreas. Plenum press, New York. London P: 1- 7.

294) Steven A and Lowe JS. Human Histology (1997). Mosby Press, London.

295) Yuanfeng H, Yufei L, Lijuan W, Hong Z, and Yu L. *Chinese Medical J* (1996) 109:819-822.

اسم الطالب : حسن فياض سمير العزاوي
اسم المشرف : الدكتور سامي المظفر
عنوان الاطروحه : دراسات كيميائية حياتية وبايولوجية على الاوليروبين وتأثيره المخفض لمستوى السكر

المستخلص

تمت دراسة المركبات الفينولية الرئيسة في ثمار أشجار الزيتون لثلاث أصناف رئيسة في العراق هي صنف لبيب ، الاشرسي ، مانزانلو بعدة طرق للاستخلاص والفصل والتنقية شملت كروماتوغرافيا الطبقة الرقيقة وكروماتوغرافيا السائل ذات الأداء العالي، حيث استخلصت ثمار الزيتون الجافة بظروف مثلى باستعمال مزيج من الميثانول : الماء بنسبة حجمية ١ : ١ أو مزيج من الايثانول:الماء بنسبة حجميه ١:٣ حيث جفف المستخلص وتم تحلليه بطريقة كروتوماتوغرافيا السائل ذات الطور العكوس ووجد بأنه لا توجد فروقاً في نوعية المركبات الفينوليه في كل هذه الأصناف الثلاثة تحت الدراسة، وإنما في تركيز هذه المركبات .

تمت دراسة تأثير الحامض والقاعدة على استخلاص مركب الاوليروبين من ثمار الزيتون حيث وجد بان هنالك تأثيرا معنويا للحامض والقاعدة على تركيز المركب اوليروبين حيث يتحرر مركب الهايدروكستايروسول لكن مستوياته تبلغ ٥٠ مرة اكبر عند التحلل بالحامض لمدة ٢٤ ساعة مقارنة بالقاعدة.

تمت دراسة الفعالية البيولوجية لمركب الاوليروبين من خلال تأثيره على تثبيط تأكسد البروتينات الشحمية ذات الكثافة الواطئة ووجد بأن له نسبة تثبيط تبلغ ٥١% مقارنة بفيتامين û . كذلك لوحظ بأة المركب الاوليروبين له كفاءة عالية كمانع للتأكسد عند استعمال مركب ازو _ بس اميدينويروبان في تحلل كريات الدم الحمراء.

تمت دراسة تأثير الاوليروبين والمركبات الناتجة عن تحلله على نمو خمسة أنواع من البكتريا المرضية حيث وجد بأة الاوليروبين كلايكوسيد ليس له تأثير على جميع أنواع البكتريا تحت الدراسة ولكن الاوليروبين أكلا يكوة والهايدروكستايروسول وحامض ألينولك والتي هي نواتج ايضية للمركب اوليروبين كلايكوسيد لها تأثيرا واضحا على تثبيط نمو جميع أنواع البكتريا .

تم إثبات تأثير الاوليروبين على خفض مستويات الكلوكوز في الدم في تجارب حيوانية باستخدام الأرانب المصابة بالسكر المحدث بمادة الالوكسان،حيث وجد بان تناول ٢٠ ملغم

يوميا من الطيروبين من قبل الأرانب المصابة بالسكر لمدة ١٦ أسبوعا يجعل مستويات السكر مقارب للحد الطبيعي .

تم إثبات تأثير تناول ٢٠ ملغم يوميا من الاوليروبين في الأرانب المصابة بفرط السكري على مستويات أشكال الدهنيات،حامض اليوريك،الهيموكلوبين المسكر وفعالية الأنزيمات المضادة التأكسد،مستويات الكلوتاثيون بالإضافة إلى مستويات مضادات التأكسد غير الأنزيمية والتي شملت فيتامين ج،ه وبيتا – كاروتية،كذلك تم قياس متغيرات حالة فائقة الأكسدة المرافقة لمرض السكري في كل من الأرانب المصابة بفرط السكر والأشخاص المصابين بالنوع الثاني من السكر بعد تناولهم جرعات محددة من مركب اوليروبين لفترات زمنية تتراوأ من ١٦ أسبوعا إلى ٦ اشهر .

تمت دراسة ارتباط هرمون الأنسولين الموسم باليود– ١٢٥ بالخلايا الليمفاوية المعزولة من دم الأشخاص المصابين بمرض السكري غير المعتمد على الأنسولين حيث وجدت نوعين من المواقع الارتباطية تمتاز الأولى بالآلفة العالية والسعة الواطئة أما الثانية فتمتاز بالآلفة الواطئة والسعة العالية من الارتباط، كذلك وجد بان عدد المواقع الارتباطية لهرمون الأنسولين تنخفض بصورة معنوية عذآ الأشخاص المصابين بالسكري مقارنة بالأشخاص الأصحاء لكن تناول ١ غم يوميا من الاوليروبين لمدة ٦ اشهر يرفع عدد المواقع الارتباطية إلى الحد شبه الطبيعي مما يوضح دور الاوليروبين في زيادة نسبة الارتباط والحفاظ على مستلمات الأنسولين من تأثير التأكسد بفعل الجذور الحرة المتكونة نتيجة التفاعلات الايضية الحاصلة في الجسم .

آA ةا الدراسة الحالية هي الأولى في الأدبيات لتوضيح تأثير الاوليروبين على جزر لنكرهانة O في خلايا بيتا المأخوذة من بنكرياس الفئران المصابة بفرط السكر المحدةE بفعل الالوكسانا حيث لوحظ بان هنالك تغيرات نسيجية في جزر لنكرهانس في الفئران المصابة بالسكري تمثلE باستمرارية تضخم الخلايا وترشح للخلايا الليمفاوية ووجود زيادة معنوية في معدل أقطار الجزر بينما تناول جرعة محددة من الاوليروبين من قبل الفئران المريضة لمدة ثلاث أسابيع أدى إلى نقصان في معدل أقطار الجزر وندرة تضخم الخلايا وبالتالي فأن الجزر تبدو طبيعية مقارنة بمجموعة السيطرة.

دراسات كيميائية حياتية وبايولوجية على الاوليبروبين وتأثيره المخفض لمستوى السكر

رسالة مقدمة إلى كلية العلوم جامعة بغداد كجزء من متطلبات نيل درجة الدكتوراه فلسفة في علم الكيمياء الحياتية السريرية

مقدمة من قبل

حسـن فياض سمير العزاوي

بكالوريوس علوم كيمياء حياتية (جامعة بغداد ١٩٨١)
ماجستير علوم كيمياء حياتية سريريه (جامعة بغداد ١٩٨٦)

بـإشراف
الأستاذ الدكتور ســـامي المظفر

تشرين الثاني ٢٠٠٤